THE WAY OF THE BOOMERANG

My Journey to ReBalance My Health with a Roadmap to Navigate Yours

JULIA HARVEY

The Way of the Boomerang
My Journey to ReBalance My Health with a Roadmap to Navigate Yours.

For more information: www.aepress.co.uk

British Library Cataloguing in Publication Data.
A catalogue record for this book is available from the British Library.

This is a work inspired by real-life events and is designed to provide an experience to readers. It is shared and sold with the understanding that the author is not engaged to render any type of psychological, medical, legal or any other kind of personal or professional advice. No warranties or guarantees are expressed or implied by the author's choice to include any of the content in this volume. The reader should always consult his or her medical, health or other professional and accredited health provider before adopting any of the suggestions in this book or drawing any ideas, inferences or practices from this book. The author shall not be liable for any physical, psychological, emotional, financial or commercial damages, including, but not limited to, special, incidental, consequential or other damages. The reader is responsible for their own choices, actions and results.

1st Edition, 1st Printing 2025
Cover and text design by Julia Harvey
Interior design by Julia Harvey
Author photos by Rachael Elliott
Edited by Gary Smailes
Imprint: Independently published by All Encompassing Press
www.aepress.co.uk
ISBN 978-1-0683331-0-1

Disclaimer

The Way of the Boomerang is not a replacement for medical intervention. I am not a doctor so the views in this book are my own. I recovered from Myalgic Encephalomyelitis ME, my health restored, and I have spent the last 36 years learning how to rebalance my health using a combination of methods and approaches. I am sharing what worked for me and what I consider to be part of my journey. Everything in this book has been tried and tested by me.

There are many routes to come back into alignment and rebalance your health and self. It's a blend. I tried as many modalities as I could to kick start my own immune system and its self-healing capacity. Some worked for me, some didn't. I went with my intuition. I had so many symptoms to overcome so this took baby steps and patience.

Please seek medical advice and attention if you are feeling acutely unwell and it is overwhelming for you. Visit your doctor to seek guidance in addition to finding a naturopath, functional medical or holistic health practitioner. Take back the reins, be the one in the know and investigate all aspects of your health. Use critical thinking skills to research and discover all the information.

Dedication

M, D, and W
Always and Forever

Acknowledgments

Gary Smailes, my editor, for respecting my words and supporting the process of streamlining what was a great amount into a manageable life and guide book.

Tracey 'TC' Smith, my long time friend, you were there when this all began at the age of twenty. Thank you for your listening ear and design help.

John Lowe from B&L Creative, for your creative support.

Rachael Elliott for your epic car brainstorms, being my most wonderful professional proofreader and photographer, thank you for being part of my journey.

Sophie Lark, your enthusiasm and encouragement has been a key part of this book birthing.

George Michael, thank you for the music, with me from the beginning and never far away as I wrote, helping me to LWP 1 *and* 2.

Luna and Honey my gorgeous ever faithful Jacks, keeping me grounded, always; reminding me to take breaks away from the screen, to walk, play and be outside in nature. Your love is weaved within these pages.

Contents

PART 2

THE SIX WAYS ROADMAP

Preface

This book has been a long time in the making and has gone through many configurations. I began to keep a diary of my ill health in that first year of 1989 and continued to do this for about five years after which it became a more intuitive fluid journalling practice. When I returned to read these notebooks, I discovered the timeline of my health journey and found similar themes amongst those pages; everything I had done was forming into six ways. Over the years, I shared these ways informally amongst friends, family, and colleagues, and later as I began teaching and lecturing, following on with clients in private practice.

The Way of the Boomerang follows me finding my way through debilitating ill health. Based within these pages is my story as I recovered from Myalgic Encephalomyelitis (ME), which began when I was twenty. In the beginning, I had no clue where to start, but I knew for sure that I was going to find out what was going on, a way to get better, discover good health alignment and restore.

In that process, I learnt about living in a holistic way and the ways of energy, frequency, and vibration nudging me further along my journey through the health fields. I became an avid researcher and investigator while exploring different types of health modalities and therapy treatments, experiencing a range of approaches, bringing gentle shifts over the months and years. It took a whole decade to heal, gradually building key components into my daily life. During those early years, I began investigating what was happening, taking back the reins and responsibility of health. I visited numerous practitioners and therapists, consultants, and doctors, some who had moved from Western medicine, some that remained firmly embedded, and others that practised integrative medicine. I explored nutrition and food intolerances and took it back to basics. I read a plethora of books, journals and research papers and, what's more, I implemented many methods into my restorative journey. Remembering that this was before the internet and Google, so everything was with greater effort and revolved around writing letters, making phone calls, and visiting the library.

My health has been at equilibrium for twenty-five-plus years; more or less. I have continued to work with these practices, ebbing and flowing, responding to curve balls when they bound in and knock me off kilter. The Way of the Boomerang is where I turn to get back in the driving seat of my health sovereignty, the very essence of who I am; my intention in writing this finally and putting it down in one volume is to share this with you too so you can find your way too.

I have experienced quite significant losses over a very short period of time, bereavement impacted my whole sense of health and self, physically dealing with pain in my body and emotionally healing and dealing.

What I was experiencing shook my foundations again.

Intuitively, I re-turned to my Six Ways and opened my ReBalancing Toolkit, they had not moved too far from me as they were always a part of my very essence since those early years. However, with all I was experiencing, I needed to start again.

This time, no one else was there next to me. It was just me. This was a different kind of exhaustion. My energy tank was empty.

I was deeply fortunate to have counselling and I am extremely grateful for these sessions and my counsellors. During one counselling session, I found myself talking about being so ill with ME, reflecting on the shock back then, I talked about approaches I had used and found myself saying.

> I'm like a boomerang, somehow I find my way back.

At that moment I realised that this book was going to be called The Way of the Boomerang, taking you through my journey of rebalancing my health back then, introducing the The Six Ways and ReBalancing Toolkit - holistic approaches, supporting body, mind and spirit. Living in balance is a daily challenge, whatever is happening in your life - it is a moment by moment dance, navigating external and internal forces. My intention within these pages is for you to know where to turn to rebalance your health in a holistic way, to have a roadmap for taking back the reins of your own health sovereignty, and becoming your own healer, once more.

Boomerang Beginnings

I was put into foster care at four days old and adopted at fourteen weeks. I arrived with massive open sores on my bottom from foster care. The doctors who ran the local surgery were extremely hands-on and used to pop in daily, to check up on me and change dressings. They were incredibly supportive. I was so fortunate and blessed to grow up with my Mum and Dad, being open to opportunities and having lovely friends; music and art were my go-to, playing the clarinet, piano and guitar, performing in plays, bands, orchestras and exploring my artistic self.

My health problems began to show around the age of two and by the age of six, I was hit with tonsillitis until thirteen. I would get one bout, recover for a couple of weeks, then get it again - it got to the point where the headmaster sent someone round to check on me at home as I was barely there. At that time in the 1980s, there was a trend to leave tonsils in, but because I was in such a rough place of perpetual illness, the doctors and my parents tracked down an ENT (ear, nose and throat) surgeon who said he would remove them. Had we known then about the overuse of antibiotics weakening my gut health, we may have left them in and dealt with what was causing the flares and infections. Had we known that tonsillitis indicates the root issue is stagnant lymph and the tonsils (plus adenoids) are the first line of the lymphatic system to drain, and tonsillectomies are just plastering over, we would have researched further. However, back then, I had missed so much schooling, we just didn't know what else to do; little did I know that it was the precursor to bringing my immune system down with a huge crash.

When asked about family history, I would always reply, '*I don't have any.*' It was at the age of around thirty when I decided to trace my birth mother. I began to wonder what health difficulties may have been in my biological family. I sat down with Mum to talk about it and, as usual, she was very supportive and encouraged me to get my original birth certificate and discover who gave birth to me.

It was all swift and simple. I sent away for my original birth certificate and discovered my birth name and my birth mother's name.

When I registered my interest in finding her through a charity called NORCAP, (National Organisation for Counselling Adoptees and Parents, now closed but amalgamated into Family Action.) I was told that she had already given her address and contact details.

So, two months after I registered, I began exchanging letters with her.

We shared letters for six months.

Those letters were very informative. I began to build a

picture of my birth story and history. We eventually met for the first time six months later.

I discovered I was conceived in Australia, this boomerang baby found her way back to being born in England, placed in foster care at four days old, finally landing with my Mum and Dad at fourteen weeks. I discovered my origins, which did help to fit more jigsaw pieces in the puzzle.

It totally made sense when I discovered I was conceived on Aussie shores as I had a love affair with Australia all my growing up years as we had very close cousins who had gone to live there.

When I began to bring this book together, I realised that the origins of my health story began here, this helped me to connect the dots to all the boomerangs.

Introduction

There's a knock on our front door. Mum is up quickly to open it. A woman with short white hair and a gentle, worn face, framed by delicate wrinkles from an ME (Myalgic Encephalomyelitis) charity enters. Her eyes, despite looking tired, shone with a resilience that told a story of great struggle. Dressed in a soft grey blouse that complemented her complexion, she uses two walking sticks for support. Every step forward is focused and takes great effort. As she gently settles into a chair, she introduces herself, revealing that she has battled ME for thirty years

"Thirty years?" Julia gulps. "Really?"

I listened to her words.

Shocked.

Thirty years.

She stayed about an hour, and when she left, Mum and I sat dumbfounded.

Why did someone come who had been ill for that length of time? Why not someone who had recovered? An individual whom I could ask medical questions, symptoms, remedies and practices.

Someone who could offer me a little bit of inspiration.

I knew how important it was to gain support from others who were also going through a similar health problem and I did connect with others who were ill with ME.

At that time, I had wanted to talk to people who were recovering or had recovered.

I wanted to see some light at the end of the tunnel. I was not looking for miracles, but I was looking for something. A kind of road map to wellness.

I think it was at that moment that the seeds for this book were sown.

As the years passed and I started to recover, I increasingly wanted to share my words and healing journey with others. I wanted to give optimism to those experiencing extreme debilitation and pain, not just with ME.

I'm sharing my Ways so you can find yours.

I am not and would never imply that I have all the answers. What I knew for sure was I was responsible for supporting my immune system back to health. I wanted to find out as much as possible, and that's what I did. I tried different treatments that some may say are a bit left of centre. Yet, I was open to investigating different modalities.

Within these pages, I am offering a window into my journey. If something resonates with you, then I am thankful. I respect where you or your loved one may be in the midst of their health journey; my endeavour is not to imply any quick fixes or rushed approaches.

Part 1 tells the story of the first five years of illness. At this time, I had no clue what was happening, but I stepped into gathering mode, reading and researching avidly. This depended on when I had the energy, when brain fog was having a clearer moment, and when headaches were taking a mini break and muscles not so lacking in energy. I took the opportunity to talk to practitioners and consultants where possible, building files of information about my health and healthcare in general from all perspectives.

I was looking at and assessing my life in a holistic way, not just the physical side of all the symptoms but also the emotional, social, environmental, and spiritual aspects. I recognised that they were all interwoven and for me to heal, I had to look at my health from all angles. This was really hard for me because I knew I hadn't brought about this traumatic health experience, but I did know that to explore things holistically, I needed to deep dive into what looking at the whole individual actually meant.

I was building a picture of how I could restore my health so I could begin living again. I discovered that the antibiotics I had taken as a very young child and throughout my younger years may be a piece of the puzzle, and that perhaps certain foods whilst not the cause of ME, could be a route to taking off the stressors and pressures from my immune system if there were intolerances. I looked at all areas with so much detail and was prepared to make changes. I knew that building quiet time into my day was absolutely crucial in managing my health and my mind.

I began to see the small beneficial impacts of the changes I was making, and I was learning a great deal about health and well-being. I was taking responsibility for my restoration; I had no other options. I found support from practitioners that I resonated with and began to integrate new methods into my daily life. In these early years, I didn't know if it was going to help me get 100% well, I knew it wasn't going to be one thing, one magic pill, one answer, but a combination of approaches: a blend.

In Part 2, I lay out the Six Ways Roadmap; included in each Way are five Way Points, these are approaches that I selected. There was no quick fix; learning about one area moved me into another phase, or I met a different practitioner or read a new book, discovering what worked well for me and what didn't. I am including only those that supported my mind, body and spirit; others that didn't work or didn't resonate, I am leaving out. You may find the same when you read them; some will appeal, whilst others, less so. Stay open to the possibilities and use the end of these sections called 'Pause' to contemplate what may be helpful for you. One may catapult your investigation into deeper territory.

Throughout the healing process, I would always turn to my five senses to assess what was happening within me, around me and to me. What am I seeing? What am I hearing? What am I smelling? What am I tasting? What am I touching?

This was most definitely the place to start for me. I also asked another very important question. What am I feeling?

What was my intuition trying to tell me? Did I have a gut reaction? What messages was I missing? More so, what was I ingesting and consuming that may have been causing congestion and inflammation?

Although I didn't realise it at the time, this twenty-year-old in 1989 was being presented with the opportunity to develop her critical thinking skills about health, life and beyond.

There is a much greater depth to all of these issues; things that are out of our control. For example:

- Soil conditions for growing food.
- Chemicals used in food and water systems.
- The quality and source of water we drink.
- Spray in our skies impacting the air that we breathe.
- Ultra processed manufactured food filled with chemicals
- Synthetic creation of materials and fabrics.

I could go on and on, these are much deeper issues with an abundance of further reading around them. Back then I began with the fundamentals, researched in greater depth and integrated new approaches as my awareness grew. These investigations materialised into my Six Ways of the Boomerang, becoming the bedrock of my life and one I have built upon over the decades.

BOOST: This Way focuses on boosting natural immunity by looking at some key components of supporting the immune system, in particular, vitamin and mineral supplements, saying goodbye to sugar, supporting the intestines with probiotics, introducing echinacea, and buying organic.

NOURISH: Relates to nourishing not only through food, for example, food combining, releasing and rotating grains and carbohydrates, hydration, clearing out chemicals and earthing. It also introduces the art of journalling as a tool for nourishing our emotional health.

SUPPORT: Examines complementary health practices; these were key for me in my health journey. I tried a plethora of different systems here; I share about: aromatherapy, reflexology, Bach Flower remedies, counselling and reiki.

COCOON: Explores routes to removing the negative drip feed from daily life; dedicated stillness, peace and quiet time, hypnotherapy, saying no, flowing into sleep, tech fasting and EMF (electromagnetic frequency). These are all routes to being more in presence and going inward.

CREATE: Exploring creativity as a well-being tool to rebalance, approaches that lift up and encourage joy; shift the focus to resonate at a higher frequency; colouring in, creating visions for a future self, making a deck of soothing cards, and elevating energy vibe through film joy.

MOVE: At the time when I was very ill, any kind of physical exercise was problematic. Physical movement set me back, so I had to find ways to move energy within and around me. This Way is related to internal and external movement. I write about practices that I did intuitively back then: affirmations, box breathing, writing letters, exploring a gentle tai chi movement and qigong exercise.

At the end of these Way Points, I include space to Pause, think of this as the slight slowing down of the boomerang as it glides on the flight path. Time for you to also slow a little as you're reading. A prompt for you to dig deeper, research further and consider, perhaps experience, or experiment.

You may want to keep a journal specifically for these prompts so that you can respond to the information and record what feels the next step forward for you.

There is no pressure to work through the book methodically. You can pick and choose any segment on its own and read through, take on board, dismiss, or pooh-pooh it – there is no real order - what resonates with you right in the present moment of reading, is where you need to be. Some of these approaches were a little wacky way back then in the early 90s; today, they have become more commonplace.

In my research and restorative process, I went on to study health at degree level and researched in much greater depth ending up teaching adult learners, here it was confirmed that health has many definitions.

To some of us, being and feeling healthy is about our physical health. As we know, our physical health impacts our emotional health and vice versa. We can be physically able and fit, yet emotionally, not feel well at all. Our environmental health can also have a huge impact on our physical health, as well as our emotional health. The same can be said for our financial, spiritual, intellectual, and social health. They are all interconnected and looking at them separately is an old paradigm.

We have to look at every area of our life – this is how we begin to return to a balanced place of health. In my experience, there are usually a variety of causes, not just one. Whatever the cause, we have to look at the greater picture.

This book is written in a creative way, encouraging you to take the reins for your own health and well-being; throughout you will undertake a wholesome review of your health so it becomes a manual for action rather than merely reading. It encourages you to critically think, review, and research. Become your own private health investigator!

Although my original story is related to my illness of ME, this book may help if you are:

- Struggling with post viral/long covid.
- Have a diagnosis of ME, CFS, Fibromyalgia.

- Tired all the time, just about coping with working, and returning home shattered.
- Feel overwhelmed and not sure which way to turn.
- Have no energy to go, do, be.
- Low in mood and experiencing mild anxiety.
- In the midst of loss and bereavement.
- Stuck, not knowing where to turn.
- Coping with food intolerances.
- Dealing with yeast infections, thrush or candidiasis.
- Supporting others as a practitioner, therapist, carer.
- Looking after a family member who is experiencing any or all of the above.

That covers a wide range, however you found me, I am so glad you're here. I invite you to step with me into The Way of the Boomerang.

Julia

Part One

Finding my way through the first few years.

Floored

The doorbell rang. I dragged myself out of bed to open the door and there she was, my ever-resilient Mum, Sheila, coming to collect me from my digs in Manchester. Always such a positive woman, five foot two inches, short dark hair, wide smile, sparkly eyes, and a sense of humour that brightened up any dire situation with a raucous laugh that was instantly recognisable, lovely hands and nails too! Being adopted, both me and my sister were her absolute life, and she completely devoted herself to us, deepened by the fact her own mother died when she was just ten years old.

I was home alone; my flat mate had gone away. For the past two days, I had been coping with some horrendous flu virus and felt much worse. A decision was made, Mum drove over to pick me up and take me back to Liverpool. We packed my small suitcase and left.

Little did I know I would never return to that flat. That was the 23rd December 1988.

I was twenty years old. I had been living and working in

Manchester for about 18 months. In the months leading up to my Mum's arrival, I felt very run down, suffering sore throats that constantly hit me like a lead balloon.

I even remember the exact date; that's how meaningful it was. If you know me well, you'll laugh right about now because yes, Julia remembers dates.

What began as 'just flu' would become a health challenge that would take over a decade to fully heal.

Holed up in bed at home, I slept. That's about all I could do. I had to lie low and let it pass through me throughout those December days.

The New Year was creeping near. A couple of days running up to it, I had been feeling a bit better. A few friends were home from university; I felt I needed to return to some kind of normality, so I pushed myself to go out and see 1989 with them. I was feeling rough when I stepped out to the house party where all the excitement was brewing. My throat was becoming inflamed by the hour, but I stuck it out. When midnight arrived, I knew this was not a great way to see in a new year. I couldn't talk.

Mum called the doctor the following day, New Year's Day. I couldn't speak and couldn't move from bed.

In walked Dr Griffiths, probably in his early thirties, glasses slipping down his nose, familiar tweed waistcoat pulling even more tightly than the last time I saw him. With his familiar nod and smile, he listened to my tale, examined my throat and diagnosed me with a suspected glandular virus.

At this point, we just thought, '*oh here we go, throat virus again.*' I had spent most of my early years with some sort of throat virus or infection. From the age of six, I had tonsillitis pretty much all the time, giving me persistent sore throats. I had my tonsils removed at the age of thirteen, but the throat problems never really left me.

After two weeks, I was still in the same situation. I would say that it had become worse. I was sleeping incessantly.

Dr Griffiths took it upon himself to come and visit me every week at this very early stage because I was too ill to leave the house. As the weeks progressed, I still had no energy. I couldn't walk far at all and couldn't sit in the waiting room. I'll never forget the feeling I felt when I wondered why he was being overly gracious with his time.

He knew something was very wrong.

Quite seriously wrong.

In this first month, we wondered why the fatigue was still with me. I did have to go and have blood tests regularly; I was very quiet when I went out. I couldn't talk because all my concentration and energy was focused on being upright. I was walking slowly like I was carrying lead in my pockets and shoes. Being out was completely overwhelming.

Little did I know it was going to get much, much worse.

All I could do was sleep; that's all I wanted to do. I was invited to friends' houses but couldn't hold myself up, so had to decline. I had to follow what my body needed. I had no choice in the matter; it was ruling the roost. It would be a long while before I could understand what was going on.

A long while.

Horizontal

I moved into the second month of being ill. Friends were phoning, but I couldn't talk to them. I had no energy to converse; I was too tired. I am having a slight out-of-body experience writing this because I could be talking about someone else. How can anyone be too tired to hold the phone and have a conversation? This was way before hands-free. Thankfully, my Mum stepped in, apologising on my behalf, and calling friends to cancel plans if they were coming over to see me. That's not great for a twenty-year-old.

I had been off work since just before Christmas and here we were in February.

> "I should be living not lying horizontal on my bed. What is going on? I should be with friends enjoying my life.

Little did I know that this was the beginning of something

that would impact me further down the line: the changing face of friendships.

There were those that understood, or at least tried to understand, and those that seemed to give me a wide berth. Interestingly, there were those that I wasn't particularly friendly with who suddenly appeared to support and give me a boost, and sometimes the ones I thought were my closest would disappear for weeks on end.

I was referred to a gastroenterologist, who diagnosed me with a severe virus, part of the glandular fever family. He signed me off for two months. My blood test results highlighted a low white blood cell count, indicating my body was fighting something, although my glandular fever tests returned negative. I was upset on leaving this appointment, but at the same time I was relieved that something had been identified. I remember very well that he told me and Mum, who came with me, that it was going to take a long time for me to recover and it could be six months more to build up my strength.

Six months!

I was stunned. Six months.

He also mentioned something called ME; though he didn't know for sure, he considered that I may have this illness.

ME, what the heck was that?

Myalgic Encephalomyelitis.

I was five months off turning twenty-one. I didn't understand what was happening, nor why had this happened to me. Everything was in slow motion.

I was in the process of stepping up for a promotion at my work in the Property Company in Manchester. I felt incredibly guilty that I couldn't fulfil this role because I knew they needed the job to be filled, so with a very heavy heart, I decided to resign from the company. I had already been off for two months and I had been signed off for another two – that's four months off work and he was guesstimating another six. I knew the situation was difficult for them; I felt very uncertain about when I was going to be back to full strength. So in conversation with Mum, I realised I had to let it go.

Was this the right decision to make?

I'll never know.

I chose that because I was thinking about the company and its needs.

I was in the dark about when I would return to full strength.

But the vibes weren't good.

Nothing was Showing Up

My low white blood cell count was being investigated, but nothing showed up. Dr Griffiths invited me to the surgery after consultation hours to discuss what was next. He was very kind; he never insisted I make an appointment and wait it out with everyone else. He knew how difficult that would be for me, so we had the morning in the diary and his receptionist would phone to say, '*Dr Griffiths can see you at 11.30 a.m. when his clinic has finished*' giving us time to get there and see him.

What a considerate thing to do.

He was not sure what was going on with me. He didn't really have a clue (by his own admittance). He had never seen this kind of lethargy before. The flu-like symptoms I was presenting were developing into something more serious: sore throat, swollen glands, severe headaches, deep fatigue, brain fog, lack of coordination, intense pain in joints and muscles which never left me, and back pain; all a collection of individual symptoms that could be anything. I was tested for lupus, Lyme disease, multiple sclerosis.

I asked Mum to buy me a journal. She returned with a bright red page-a-day diary from WHSmith. Smiths' was our go-to or Woolworths (Ah, Woolies!)

Writing had always been a constant companion of mine; from a very early age I would write and colour in, and this time seemed like no exception. I used the space to compose my thoughts, get them on the page and out of my head. I was nearly twenty-one and dealing with a severe virus. When I read my words, I feel very sorry for the young woman before me.

Yet even then, I began writing this very first mantra to myself, inspired by Monty Python.

'*Always look on the bright side of life.*'

I needed some hope.

I would doodle this mantra all over the page. Writing out lines like I used to get in school. This time, it didn't say, '*I must not talk in class.*'

This time, I wrote it out, line after line, after line, after line.

Always look on the bright side of life
Always look on the bright side of life
Always look on the bright side of life
Always look on the bright side of life
Always look on the bright side of life

I was desperately trying to keep my emotions UP. I could feel my active twenty-year-old life fading. You know how you can reduce the opacity of a photograph? Well, that's how it was beginning to feel. It wasn't sharp anymore. I couldn't see what was next. My plans were losing their opacity and were becoming translucent.

My friends were getting on with their lives, finishing their degrees, studying for masters, making new friends, finding boyfriends, falling in love, getting engaged, getting married, travelling, moving to new countries.

I felt like I was waiting at traffic lights, waiting for the amber light... only green wasn't coming any time soon.

I wasn't even twenty-one yet.

For the next three months, I didn't write much, though I continued to see Dr Griffiths. Yet due to severe ill health, I was sleeping for most of this time, coping with all the symptoms I felt like I had some sleeping disease.

I did pick up a pencil and began to sketch randomly whenever I felt I had an ounce of oomph. Art and craft had always been medicine for me. Here was a small seed of joy. An HB pencil and a plain white piece of paper in a sketchbook. I didn't have much strength to hold the pencil for long but here and there, I would try to doodle, a heart, a bird, a dog's face, a flower, just something.

Falling Deep into Lethargy

The weeks passed and before I knew it, I had been ill for six months; my health had fallen into deep fatigue and lethargy. Any exertion was painful, and it all had to be planned, such as taking a shower or visiting the toilet.

I was beginning to feel like a recluse. I still hadn't heard the words ME again; my diagnosis at this point was post-viral fatigue syndrome. I began to lose the sense of what was normal; everyone was carrying on with their lives and of course, why wouldn't they?

I had the inklings of fear writing in my journal;

> “is this normal for me now? Will I ever be well again? When will I be able to get back to my life?

People cared but they didn't understand, and it was hard to expect them to understand because I didn't know... this was new to me too.

What I knew for sure, and what Mum knew for sure, I was not making this up.

Mum was my one saving grace. She knew I was seriously not well; she believed me. She was Chief Supporting Office and El Grande Protector. She is weaved throughout my back-to-health story because I deeply believe, had she not been the kind, wonderful, caring, funny woman she was, I would not have recovered.

Mum's the Word

I could write an entire book about my Mum, Sheila. She was always there for me, a rock, a support and a boundary to the outside world.

In the first instance, let me just say:

1. Mum did not want me to stay at home with her, as some people thought.
2. She wasn't 'mollycoddling' me (that word really began to annoy me).
3. She knew I was very ill, and she was not protecting a hypochondriac.
4. She knew it wasn't yuppie flu as the mainstream media coined it and people would say.

She faced all these comments from people; family, friends, members in her community, and she bravely batted them away, knowing within her heart that this was something she didn't want to engage in. She knew she didn't have to prove anything to anyone.

In the early stages of finding things out together, it was always me and her. I had just moved away and was suddenly back after two years. Dad was working and very focused on his new business, he cared deeply from the sidelines but felt helpless. Mum knew from the word go that something was wrong; this was not 'just' flu, and she had to fight hard to be heard. She would always accompany me if I had an appointment but gave me space. She never pushed her way in but still nurtured my independence, which was fading. With Dad being away all day and on business trips, it ended up that Mum would be the one taking me to consultations, new treatments, therapies. I would often need her help in the early days to reflect on the words from practitioners and consultants as my brain fog was a key symptom.

She was a sponge, just like me, soaking up all the information we could find. People would often contact us and tell us about their sister, brother, wife, father, husband, daughter, son, etc, who were ill and she would always be on the end of the phone talking to people, sharing insights and ways that I was progressing.

She wasn't that particularly well herself with high blood pressure. I am sure that my illness added so much more stress on her; we talked a lot about this and she told me it didn't, but I'm not sure. She was stoic; she got me through daily with her humour and her '*sense of ridiculous*' as she coined herself. She always phoned me when she was out shopping, asking if I could think of anything else to buy; many years later, she told me that she phoned whilst out to check if I was okay, to hear my voice and to reassure herself that I wasn't flat out having fainted or fallen. She would also feel so guilty leaving me. This was in the days before mobile phones, so the supermarket phone had a real purpose in the 90s.

The devotion of my Mum was second to none, she was a lioness when it came to cub protection. No one could say a bad word or anything negative against me, which I see now could have been problematic as she was gently fierce (and she got fiercer in later life). It was beautiful to see her joy after my sister's three daughters arrived. I wanted her to go and feast on these beautiful baby girls and spend time with them, seeing them grow, so she would leave plates of food in the freezer for me and Dad to defrost. She had the most wonderful relationship with her three granddaughters; they had a bond that couldn't be broken, even after she passed away five years ago, she is still so rooted in their lives and within her great-grandchildren. She passed away having four of them, and there have been another five since she died. She lived for her family and was deliriously happy with such joy everyday hearing about them. Her Sheila 'isms' continue on.

She wrote her own book called My Girl and Me; the afterword is an excerpt of these words. Much of our story overlaps; having her in my book feels so right. I know that I would not be here today were it not for her.

I am beyond grateful for her devotion and dedication.

The Southport Healer

I was now dealing with continuous back pain, muscle aches, deep fatigue and headaches. I was in limbo land. I felt like I had landed in a new land at the top of The Magic Faraway Tree by Enid Blyton. It was completely alien to me. I was living a life that I didn't recognise.

Around this time, someone recommended that I see a woman in Southport, who was known to be a healer of sorts. She was '*into alternative medicine*' we were told.

I had no knowledge of alternative medicine.

Mum had no clue, either.

We were both immersed in Western allopathic medicine and anything off-centre was a bit quacky. It all felt weird to me. Yet, I was open to anything that may help me begin to get well again. Any perspective of what was going on was needed.

I found myself in her examining room in my bra and knickers (feeling very heavy and bulky because of immobility). I am being prodded and poked. She felt all my pressure points, front and back, examined my eyes, mouth, and she checked my spine in great detail. There wasn't really any explanation. I didn't feel part of this examination.

I felt cold, exposed and yukky.

But what she did say - and this was the first time I had heard anyone speak about anything that was different - she asked me not to wear any brass or plastic jewellery. She also asked me to avoid wearing tampons and suggested that I stop eating wheat.

This summed up the consultation.

It felt very 'out there' and I wasn't sure what I achieved, but she was the first individual to suggest ditching the tampon and exploring nutrition as a way back to wellness. That was it. I never saw her again.

Yet, a seed was planted.

Turning Twenty-One

Seven months in and here comes my twenty-first birthday. What a complete downer. I couldn't go anywhere; my health and energy level dictated what I could and couldn't do.

Mum came up trumps again and organised an open house party where people dropped in to see me. This way, I could manage seeing people in small numbers rather than everyone arriving at the same time, which would have tired me out completely.

Fab food from Mum, yet again, her old favourites came out: tiffin, peanut crunchies, florentines, pavlova, birthday cake, and all manner of scrummy yumminess. She really went to town to make my twenty-first feel special. Anyone who grew up with me knew of her peanut crunchies, florentines and tiffin; we all adored them. Later on I would discover that all these foods were impacting my symptoms. Yummy nonetheless!

During those few hours when friends and family popped

in, there was talk of new friendships, boyfriends, engagements, weddings, babies, travelling and jobs.

Putting on a happy face, I always wanted to hear people's good news but inside my heart was hurting as I couldn't see any of this for myself. It was at this particular point that my hands and wrists became inflamed and I noticed a fungal infection starting in my fingernails.

Knowing what I know now, this was a sign of a more serious problem that was lurking in my gut.

The Dreaded DHSS

September arrived and a letter landed on my doorstep from the DHSS, the Department of Health and Social Security as it was known then. I was being asked to attend a medical in Liverpool City Centre as they questioned my incapacity to work. The DHSS were formed in 1968, disbanded in the early 90s, then reformed as the Department for Work and Pensions in 2001.

Anxiety hit me. Getting myself ready to go, being driven, parking, walking and waiting for this medical was so difficult, but it had to be done.

Thankfully, Mum also came with me. I don't know what I would have done had she not been the type of mum she was. Always right by my side, walking the journey with me. This must have been so very difficult for a woman in her mid-fifties to witness her twenty-one-year-old daughter going through all of this.

I was called into the examination room. The doctor, who was elderly, didn't even make eye contact with me and conducted an extremely poor and uncommunicative consultation. Compared to Dr Griffiths, who was lovely, I couldn't quite understand why this man didn't want to know what was happening. I left feeling very demoralised. A week later, I received a letter from the DHSS, who declared after my medical, that according to this doctor, I was '*fit to work*' and it would be of '*therapeutic value*'.

I was stunned, we all were.

On visiting Dr Griffiths to discuss the outcome of the letter he was appalled. How could the DHSS doctor make this conclusion? He had spent not even ten minutes with me, in comparison to Dr Griffiths, who saw me weekly for nine months. It undermined his own appraisal of my illness and he decided he was going to appeal this decision. He felt I was not in any way fit to return to work.

After about four weeks, I received a letter in response to the appeal.

'A report has been received from your doctor and it has been decided that a further examination is not necessary at present.' Dr R L

Thank goodness I had Dr Griffiths on my side. I heard so many horror stories of doctors not believing their patients and letting them flounder. I was very thankful and still am to this day.

> I'm going to try to get back to the Old Julia.

Little did I know that the '*Old Julia*' would not be seen again.

Homeopathy

Soon after my birthday, I heard about a homeopathic doctor called Dr Bird, who practised in Liverpool. He was a trained medical practitioner but had decided to move into the field of homeopathy. I didn't know anything about homeopathy, but I chatted to Mum about the idea. We got a book from the library and thought, '*what have I to lose*?' We made an appointment to see him.

Homeopathy is a system of complementary medicine in which ailments are treated by very small doses of natural substances that in larger amounts, would produce symptoms of the ailment. Like treats like. It is a form of vibrational essence, with the tincture containing the essence of the substance. The first appointment was a huge gathering of information. This is where my first introduction to a holistic approach began because I had to fill in a form that was approximately twelve pages long, asking so many different questions, relating from my digestion, amalgam fillings, to the texture of my poo and how often I had my period and the different styles of bleed. I had never encountered anything like this, and it felt pretty weird to be answering, but this was the first person enquiring about All of Me.

I had so many symptoms I think he was overwhelmed on what to focus upon first. At this point, I was eight months into feeling so poorly. In this first appointment, he suggested that I take vitamin E for my hair, skin and nails. My illness was so clear to see - manifesting in my hair, which was lank, limp and stringy.

I wouldn't be surprised if Dr Bird went to have a strong brandy after seeing me. I was a complete mess, although I was feeling a little uplifted. He was the first practitioner who really delved deeply; he knew I was genuinely ill and not putting it all on.

It was now nearly September; I desperately wanted to feel better. I had a dream of studying art at college, but I was just not well enough to go, so at this point, I could only dream and visualise '*Julia as artist.*' I was feeling more and more down about my health, despite seeing Dr Bird, I was trying to figure out how I could turn a corner.

Spot Explosion

Dr Bird had given me a remedy; the aim, he explained, was to get rid of toxins and poisons in my body.

'*They may make you feel more run down*,' shared Dr Bird.

After four days of taking the homeopathic medication, I was getting a reaction, more flu-like symptoms - this wasn't pleasant. It really felt like I had gone back a few months and this was making me worse. Was it worth it? About two weeks later, I developed a huge spot explosion on my temples.

Big boils were oozing pus and blood.

Delightful.

They were itchy and driving me nuts. They were exploding on my pillow every night, so I had to go to bed with gauze and micropore dressings to avoid aggravating them. It was so upsetting.

I was not feeling well; my throat was sore again and inflamed. I went to see Dr Griffiths, who was shocked at the reaction to the homeopathic remedy. Although he never discouraged me from exploring all possibilities, he was worried at this reaction and called to speak with Dr Bird.

He prescribed penicillin for my sore throat, which I took. Years later and more research and experience tell me that I should have stayed well away from antibiotics because further down the line, I discovered something pivotal in the investigation for supporting and healing my immune system.

The toxins were coming out of my body - the blood and pus were being evicted - dramatically, but nonetheless, the crap was escaping. I also was prescribed antibiotic cream for my exploding spots, which I used.

I wasn't put off from homeopathy, but I had to try to alleviate the outpouring; it didn't feel like it was working.

> “ I would really like a change in scenery, a different atmosphere, I'm fading here, but wherever I go, my body comes with me and although the air may be lovely and sunny, my body is in tatters.

Ain't Giving Up

After a few months of seeing Dr Bird, the oozing spots had calmed down a little but there was still gunk coming out and scarring my skin. He gave me marigold tablets for the next consultation to help soothe the affected temples and boost my immune system. At this point, I didn't really know much about marigold, but I took it upon myself to research the basic information about it - also known as calendula, it has anti-inflammatory properties when the dried petals are infused with a carrier oil such as coconut oil or sweet almond oil.

I was in shock. I could not believe that I was still very ill. It all seemed so unreal, yet it truly was very real. Nonetheless, through all this, I carried on trying to find as much information as I could, but it was challenging because I didn't have any definitive diagnosis, I was just told continuously that I had post-viral fatigue, with no answers as to how to get anywhere with that, or what had caused it. This also proved difficult because it was before the internet where you could quickly and simply search for specialised topics and up would pop a selection of scientific studies, library held documents, health and wellness website; I had to go to the library or look through the Yellow Pages.

Connecting Dots

Around this time, Mum bumped into the mother of Martin Lev; we used to know him and his brother as they went to the same school as us. Being an actor Martin was also very ill with ME. I remember him starring as Dandy Dan in the film Bugsy Malone in 1976. He suffered the debilitating effects of ME for seven years, and it was through this health challenge he founded The ME Action Campaign along with Sue Finlay and Clare Francis. His mum told him about me, and he sent a selection of leaflets. They were jam packed full of information that was so revolutionary at the time - I still have them - they were a complete game changer for me. I still hadn't had an official diagnosis, but all paths led here. This info pack was priceless.

1. **The ME Hypothesis**: This was a radical thing for The ME Action Campaign to do and they did it with caution. They realised that it would be controversial to publish their hypothesis/theory

but felt that holding back the ideas may be far more damaging for those coping with such debilitating ill health. All ideas were on the table. This was before any proof of some of these ideas. However, any line of scientific enquiry had to start somewhere - with a hypothesis, an idea, then tested, proved or disproved. It allows and encourages discussion and debate from all experts rather than listening to just one narrative. Science is a word that denotes 'knowledge': originally from Old French and from Latin *scientia*, from scire 'know'. Through observation, experimentation, evaluation, research, discussion, debate and integration this is the meaning behind science. 'The Science' is not definitive.

2. **ME Information for Employers**: This was a summary from a research paper from The Journal of Society of Occupational Medicine 1988, which discussed the course of twelve patients with post-viral fatigue syndrome following a return to work, all active people, mostly in their late-twenties and early-thirties.
3. **ME A Guide for the Non-Sufferer**: This was hugely helpful to have as I could give this to family and friends, it gave an overview of what I was feeling. This was before blogging or videos, so it was always difficult to succinctly share how I felt and how ME was defined.
4. **ME Information for Doctors**: This was designed to provide a concise, easily understandable background about diagnosis, typical symptoms,

research, what tests could be ordered, prognosis, and GP management.

5. **Diet Factsheet**: This was a generic information leaflet but introduced some basics for avoidance, e.g., processed foods, refined carbohydrates, alcohol, coffee, tea, sugary drinks, fried foods, wheat, dairy and sugar.
6. **Candida Factsheet**: Introducing and going into more details about candida, treatments, processes, dietary dos and don'ts, and anti-fungal medication.
7. **Probiotics Factsheet**: A great intro to the bowel/large intestine and how it contains millions of bacteria and other organisms such as fungi and viruses. Some are potentially dangerous if they get out of control and are held in check by 'good bacteria.' Differences between probiotics and prebiotics and where to find them.
8. **Stress, Meditation and Relaxation Factsheet**: This goes into more detail about the effects of stress, and how prolonged stress can have real physical effects, becoming very damaging on the holistic health of an individual.
9. **Vitamin and Mineral Factsheet**: A great introduction to vitamins and minerals, recommended daily allowances, nutrients, binders, fillers, tablet, capsule, liquid, plus tests for deficiencies.
10. **Allergy and Food Intolerance Factsheet**: this outlined what an allergy was and how that differed to an intolerance, allergy testing, chemical

sensitivity, causes, enzymes, bugs, and it introduced the concept of an Elimination Diet.

The information that Martin sent me had a huge effect. I had never heard about any of these possible contributing factors on health, and it opened up a new investigation portal for me. Martin searched for a way of handling his condition and set up a charity that went on to help thousands of individuals.

Devastatingly Martin died in March 1992 in tragic circumstances. I will be forever grateful and thankful for his actions to establish a variety of discussions about holistic health and ME. After Martin's death in September 1993, The ME Action Campaign changed its name and logo to Action for ME and Chronic Fatigue, which resulted in complaints as '*chronic fatigue*' is a symptom distinct from ME and CFS, (chronic fatigue syndrome.) It then changed its name in 1993 to Action for ME.

Sweet Enough

Dr Bird rang to discuss my blood test results. He said that I had a mal absorption of the small bowel, low cholesterol and high sugar count. Here '*sugar*' was mentioned again to me. I had never ever thought about sugar within a gut context, although mainstream refer to it in relation to weight gain, diabetes and possible later causation for coronary heart disease. I hadn't ever read or heard anything about the negative health implications of sugar from a gut perspective and yet here I was finding out this information, only to find that one of the information sheets from Martin Lev and The ME Action Campaign was about sugar and how it could be impacting on the immune system and releasing toxins back into the bloodstream. More so, it can be a source of increase related to a yeast in the bowel called *Candida Albicans*. I had a feeling that this was going to become much more relevant to me. This was the beginning of a very long stretch of time where I would embark upon a new way of eating to eliminate the overgrowth in my system.

Around this time, I had another allergy and intolerance test, the foods that appeared again showing sensitivities were lamb, soya, rye – upon talking this through with Dr Bird, we decided that I continue not to eat the following: lamb, turkey, veal, duck, pineapple, apples, oranges, bananas, nuts, cherries, currants, white cabbage, spinach, mushroom, wheat flour, wheat bran, yeast, soya, rye. At this point, I began to read The Yeast Connection by Gill Edwards, not knowing what a huge impact this would have.

> “ What on earth am I consuming.

The Food Relationship

On my next visit to Dr Bird, he suggested I have an allergy test called a Vega Test - I had no clue what was going on but was open to discovering if there were any intolerances with food that may turn up. I had an inkling there was, but I didn't really know.

In asking Dr Bird about the Vega Test, he told me it was a quick and simple process, testing for hundreds of substances and ingredients by reading the body's electromagnetic response. Being non-invasive and painless, it uses the body's sensitive electromagnetic system against various substances to generate a report. This was way beyond anything I had ever heard of, but it was the first time anyone had introduced me to the idea that our body was electrical and magnetic. Here, a seed was planted, and I began to reflect upon what was happening in my body.

The foods that were raised as sensitive on this day were turkey, duck, veal, lamb, pineapple, apples, oranges, bananas, cherries, nuts, currants, spinach, white cabbage, mushrooms, yeast and wheat.

I was very shocked at this list - so was Mum!

Dr Bird suggested I do my best to cut these out of my eating routine. That was a shock. However, looking back, I realised that this was the first time anyone had mentioned that certain foods could be impacting and disturbing my digestion and consequently causing inflammation and congestion.

Mum and I took this seriously; it was the first time anyone had given us a smidgeon to go on and we were on a mission. Led by her, we talked about the foods I could replace, and I began to cut things out gently. I didn't want to do it in one big leap. I phased it in over a week or so. My sister and Mum would spend hours on the phone talking about recipes. My sister, with a teaching degree in Home Economics, is a complete whizz in the kitchen, she can make a four course meal out of three ingredients! Not long after stopping yeast and wheat, aka bread and pasta, I developed huge painful ulcers in my mouth. I didn't understand what was going on, my body felt like it was constantly failing me; every step forward, I was thrust back two.

I investigated the possible cause of mouth ulcers; I discovered that they could be due to a response to bacteria in the mouth, sensitivity to foods containing acids, an intolerance to gluten, or lack of essential vitamins and minerals (B12, zinc, iron, folate). All of this felt wrapped up in what I was stopping eating, again as though my body was pushing out what it didn't want.

Not Fun Fungus

I was seeing Dr Bird every four weeks for a homeopathic appointment; he seemed to be doing his utmost to support my body system into healing. However, there were just too many symptoms, and it was extremely overwhelming for me and, I am sure, for him. Yet he never gave up.

I was beginning to.

We discussed Candida Albicans more thoroughly, although we didn't know whether that was part of the problem. Nonetheless, we talked about the possibility of beginning an antifungal remedy. The main premise of this would be eliminating my body of more toxins within the bowel. I hesitated because I generally was feeling so incredibly unwell. My lethargy and fatigue were at an all-time high and my spots were continuously spewing out gunk; I really didn't want to see what else would happen. I didn't want to add anything to an already diseased body. I was very weak.

However, when I began to piece together the information about candida and antibiotics, lightbulbs were sparking, and I recognised a connection between my early years of tonsillitis and what was presenting for me. I continued to see Dr Bird but realised that relying on one main route was not the way forward for me; I wanted to explore other options. I decided to take some time away from homeopathy and explore other modalities.

Dr Bryceson London 1990

Dr Griffiths wrote a letter for an appointment with a consultant called Dr Bryceson in Wimpole Street, London at the Centre for Tropical Diseases. Looking back on it now, I am not sure how we found out about him. I think he may have been related to gastroenterology and I can't find any records to show who he was. We were grasping at straws in the hope that he may be able to offer any insight. I have a recollection that Dr Griffiths had heard that he was seeing patients who had ME. He had read all my reports, dismissed any of the homeopathic findings and summed up to Mum and me.

"A little swimming or gentle exercise may help. Julia should embark on antidepressants to help with sleeping. Have more blood tests and revisit in two to three months."

He was very cold and distant. I came away from this appointment feeling very despondent and low. Is this all he could say? Antidepressants for sleeping were not a solution for me at all, I didn't want any synthetic chemicals in my body. Swimming and gentle exercise were not on my radar at this point, it took all my energy to get up, shower and do my best to proceed through the day.

> “Waking up I feel I have a tonne of lead strapped to my shoulders and legs, finding it difficult to walk – my legs are stuck in mud. Anything that I do during the day, takes so much energy from me. Feels like I’m in a dark tunnel, I can’t bear to see how my life has changed. Not the person I was but I will get through this somehow.

Dr Downing London 1991

I was introduced to the book Why ME; a guide to combating post viral illness by Dr Belinda Dawes and Dr Damien Downing in 1991. It built upon the information I devoured from The ME Action Campaign. There was a clinic in South London and after discussing in great detail with Mum and Dad, finding out costs, tests and trains, we decided to take a leap and make an appointment.

It was a novel approach because they were a private clinic but by this time, I had been ill for three years. I was floundering with so many symptoms and no tests were being done on the NHS. The whole experience of getting there was challenging in its own right as I had to get the train to London. I thankfully was able to stay at my sister's and, in small increments, I was able to get to the clinic. As with any exertion, I always had to factor in the time to recover because everything exhausted me.

Before the appointment, I had to complete an even longer questionnaire than Dr Bird's homeopathic consultation form. This was digging deeper, revealing everything about me, questions I had never been asked before; about perfumes I wore, what products were used in the house, my reaction to smells, if I had ever been exposed to chemicals, plus the usual of what my periods were like, stool samples, dietary choices, etc.

They meant business. There and then, I knew everything was connected, I didn't know how but I was going further into this than before.

That first appointment was where Dr Downing assessed my answers, working out what to do next. In the first instance, he realised that coming all the way to London was not going to be helpful for me, so he told me that he wanted me to see him in York; this way, Mum could drive and come with me, thereby being able to stop and be supported. He talked in great detail about candida overgrowth, chemical sensitivities, cell renewal and vitamin and mineral supplementation in a way that I had never heard anyone talk in this much detail before, especially talking about the immense value of vitamin C, as well as the huge benefits of vitamin D3 along with vitamin K2; he was the first to mention endocrine disruptors and again, the impact of antibiotics.

I was sent to a clinic nearby to embark on a series of blood and sweat tests. From these test results, I was encouraged to take a very high-quality multivitamin, buffered vitamin C in powder form that I could regulate quite clearly, zinc and magnesium at night. This is where I was first introduced to The Allergy Research group and their range of supplements. He also recommended that I have separate intravenous administrations. In those days, this was seen as quite radical, but I had really nothing to lose and everything to gain.

Looking back now, this kickstarted my innate self-healing capabilities. Again, this is my experience and I'm not claiming this would be the case for everyone, however, from having these intravenous injections, my immune system began to wake up and my natural immunity began to function. They were not the easiest of injections as they took a couple of hours, but as usual, Mum was right there, by my side, we'd chat, laugh and talk about all sorts of different things. I went on to have them every three months over the next couple of years along with supplementation in between.

Dr Collins Manchester 1992

Dr Downing wasn't available for my next appointment, so it was suggested I see his colleague Dr Collins, who had a practice in Manchester. That was another step in the right direction for me to manage the process of these appointments because it was counterproductive to go all that way to London or York and be completely washed out for a week. Manchester was very appealing; once again, Mum could drive and attend wherever necessary.

I was still struggling when I went to see him in May of 1992; I had another candida test and a range of blood tests. I was beginning to understand where I was going with all this and realised my immune system had taken such a beating from all the antibiotics throughout my life so far that I knew I had to commit to an anti-candida way of eating seriously. This was big. A huge change: I had begun to limit sugar but wasn't sure if it was helping me because I seemed to feel much worse but knew I had to do it - it seemed a tangible way of taking stressors off my immune system.

There were also other significant areas that Dr Collins helped me:

1. He said I had to have Good Quality Rest Time for one to two hours a day. Seems a strange thing to say to someone who was exhausted most of the time, but what he was affirming was the quality. To remove sound stimuli from my nervous system: no TV, radio, or distractions from 4 p.m. to 6 p.m. daily. He also wanted me to get to sleep by 10 p.m.
2. He suggested I step up my commitment to the anti-candida way of eating No yeast, sugars, mushrooms, cheese, pickles etc. in any way at all. My bloating may not necessarily be because of the candida overgrowth as it is a symptom of ME, an immune dysfunction, but we needed to see if it was.
3. In addition to vitamin and mineral supplementation, include omega 3 and 6. In particular, Mega GLA and Mega EPA, plus to continue with intravenous vitamin C.
4. He did not want me to engage in any physical cardiovascular exercise. Whatever was manageable, small steps.

Following all the steps from Dr Collins, being very seriously committed to an anti-candida diet, I took small steps forward and was beginning to see shards of light peeking through. I continued this way for a couple of years until I needed to review.

Harald Gaier Naturopath
London 1994

I was seeking new ways of exploring much further how to get my immunity and system back into balance and discovered Harald Gaier, who practised from The Nutri Centre in Hale Crescent, London. Seeing him helped me to further support my immunity and food intolerances. He added a new perspective with gut permeability tests, which then took me down the road to the gut microbiome. I didn't and don't have a diagnosis of irritable bowel but it had taken a huge hit with the overgrowth of the yeast organism Candida Albicans.

The balance in my gut was very much out of sync; therefore, I needed to address this with high-dose probiotics again. IBS has gone through so many different name changes, and it is generally considered to include bloating, discomfort after food, bowel rumblings, stomach pain, mucus in stools, possibly constipation as well as diarrhoea, decreased concentration, fatigue, lethargy and poor quality of sleep. I was still encountering some of these problems, so other things were at play. I found the support from Harald Gaier at this next phase of my healing journey a very crucial component in functional medicine.

Don't ask me where this inner warrior strength came from, but this twenty-five-year-old just knew instinctively and intuitively that she could find her way out of this.

Onwards and Upwards

My progress continued to move upward in a positive direction. I carried on eating the way I had been and built upon the foundations of research. I wasn't doing one thing but a blend of approaches. The Ways I will introduce to you in part two, have their roots here, from boosting immunity, nourishing body and mind, cultivating peace and quiet through stillness, seeking support from complementary and alternative health practitioners, creativity to shift the focus and finding a way to integrate movement.

I was able to study and train to be a counsellor on a part time basis.

I began to turn a corner.

I applied to university, where I studied an honours degree in Health. I could just about manage the commitment and all the extra research and prep, and I could now work one and a half days in a health food shop. I had to devote and balance my life to do all this. I didn't have a 'student' social experience because I had to plan my days and couldn't take anything for granted.

I married at twenty-eight. We had met through our ill health, and looking back now, we were catalysts for each other, propelling us forward in our health investigation, wellness quest and supporting one another in those early days. Unfortunately, we divorced six years later, however, his knowledge and experience helped me hugely. After graduating at twenty-nine, I secured a lecturing position for adult students at a Further Education College, teaching health and social care. I began sessional teaching hours at the university where I had just graduated.

My health was shifting. I was responding to all of the healing.

Recently, I was listening to an interview on the radio, with quite a well-known woman who also had ME for many years (she described herself as a sufferer, I dislike the word sufferer and didn't want to use that for myself). She was talking about her own ill health with ME, how she had been so ill, coping with the day-to-day ME symptoms. She explained:

'I have never ever met anyone who has got well. Anyone who has ME will always have it – they'll either be in remission or recuperating.'

I don't class myself in either of those groups. I'm always balancing.

It dawned on me, there and then, that people who have been ill with ME and recover don't tend to look back to share their story or their ways through. They have spent too much time being unwell with so many challenging symptoms; after they recover, they want to embrace the life they have. Plus, they have to play catch up with being well, feeling healthy, with relationships, families, careers, and experiences.

I realised that was me.

I didn't want to go back to look at this very upsetting and distressing time. I didn't want to stay in this past reality.

I got stuck into my career and my life. In my thirties and forties, I was always focused on my health and creating balance, especially when the curve balls came and boy, they came. I was always supportive and helpful if anyone wanted to speak to me about it and seek me out. While working as a counsellor, lecturer, and holistic health practitioner in private practice, I began to share The Six Ways and supported family, friends, students, clients, and colleagues to discover their own ReBalancing Toolkit, as well as delivering presentations in educational, business, communal and therapeutic settings. I realised finally that what helped me was helping them and that is where this flight path takes us next.

I could spend many more pages talking about the negative aspects of my health problem, there were many low points in this back to health journey, it took me a decade to get back on track, but I know that staying in the past isn't productive, nor is just recounting the negativity, so it's time for me to introduce The Six Ways Roadmap.

Part Two

The Six Ways Roadmap

Here I introduce you to The Six Ways, where I encourage you to build your ReBalancing Toolkit. As you read through each Way you'll find five Way Points held within, there are thirty in total. There are times to *Pause*, jot down notes, research further, discuss, experience and experiment. You don't have to do everything all at the same time, you can consider one approach, although you may find you want to connect a few together; ask yourself - what do I need today?

Not only is Part 2 a further dive into my ME health journey, it is an invitation for you to contemplate how to rebalance your health and self, your body, mind and spirit.

Experiment with these Six Ways, give them time to settle and see what works for you daily, weekly, and monthly. You don't have to use them in order, the aim is to build your own signature prescription. You'll add and subtract more of your own, choose what you want to focus upon in the here and now; make it your roadmap.

- What feels relevant?
- What is your intuition trying to tell you?
- What is your gut reaction?
- What messages are you missing because you aren't in the driving seat?
- What are you ingesting and consuming that may be causing congestion and inflammation?
- Are you giving your power away?

The time is most definitely now to develop critical thinking skills about your health. If not now, when?

The first Way

Boost

to help or encourage (something) to increase or improve;
a range of measures to boost, e.g. health.
to amplify (an electrical signal).

This Way explores how I began to help my immune system, thereby assisting my natural immunity.

I had learnt so much from the consultants and practitioners I had seen plus all the information I had read from The ME Action Campaign, books, articles and research. It prompted me to really look into the overuse of antibiotics and implications of yeast overgrowth, which led me down the path of vitamins, minerals and probiotics. This was a huge area for me because of how depleted my immune system was back then and I had to support it as best as I could. I began to discover that there were herbal remedies to turn to and that the overuse of chemicals in fruits and vegetables on a grander scale were messing up the quality of the soil.

Boosting my immune system's innate self-healing capabilities was the first place I started. I offer this Way here for you to contemplate.

B: Vitamins & Minerals

This is a considerable area for investigation. For over thirty-six years I have looked at how I can stay balanced using preventative approaches and holistic applications. I always turned to an original remedy or something that nature offered because I didn't want any chemical to overshadow my immune system's innate capacity to heal, restore and protect. I felt that a chemical component would initiate consequences and knock-on effects within my whole body system, one that interferes with my innate healing ability, plus the side effects from synthetic pharmaceuticals are vast.

I learnt a great deal about immunity and the power of my immune system. Vitamin and mineral supplements were crucial for boosting my immune system. I used ethical sources with the lowest allergen level and the ones with the purest vitamin content. Supermarket brands were out the window - this was either independent health store territory or specialised companies by practitioner only.

I have often been asked why you can't get your vitamins and minerals from food?

We can, we do; however, if our immune system is compromised and weak or struggling with added stress, we often need a boost from a reputable source. There is also the other impact of chemicals in the soil and water systems, sprayed onto source food, which depletes the actual food item, along with whether it is grown locally or from across the world when it will lose nutrients in transit. These are greater issues than I'm going to cover here. Go with your gut instinct on what you feel you need at this time.

I have shared about my experiences of having vitamin supplements injected intravenously when I was slap bang in the throes of ill health. This course of treatment is quite a commitment, but bear in mind that my immunity was extremely debilitated. Having a push of supplements directly would help kick my immune system into self-healing.

Whatever my body did not need, I urinated out.

I attended several sessions spaced out over twelve weeks. I discovered very early on that restoring my innate capacity to heal my immune system was key.

Creating the right environment around me that seemingly is never talked about, providing the nutrients, and addressing emotional triggers help to release the stressors on our body and mind. This is the foundation of epigenetics, first introduced by Dr Bruce Lipton. His research concludes that it is our environment that switches on our genes.

It also linked me to germ versus terrain theory. Germ theory suggests that we are susceptible to germs and therefore we must always be on the lookout for new germs. It states that it is the germ itself that makes us ill and sick, while terrain theory suggests that it is our own body's system that can and will block the germs because of the state of health we are in, which is why some people will get viruses and others won't during a flu season. There is another discussion that flu season is a depletion of vitamin D3 because the sun retreats in the northern hemisphere. vitamin D3 trials were based on research for treating rickets in children, which is why only 400 iu (international units) per day is the recommended daily allowance compared to the current research of 4000 iu a day. That's something to reflect upon.

Our natural immune system has often been brushed aside; we see ourselves as invincible and capable of coping with everything and anything. Or we seek out solutions that are chemically and synthetically created. It is not generally taught to us about the healing capacity of our immune system, but here's the thing: when you cut yourself what happens? When you break a bone, what happens? Our cells are continuously regenerating.

In my initial explorations, it was vitamin C in its loose form ascorbic acid, that I turned towards. It is one of the vitamins that has been researched and trialled and has so many benefits:

- Protects your body from getting infections.
- Repairs wounds.
- Acts as an antihistamine for asthma, sinus, colds, flu.
- Lowers blood pressure.
- Dilates blood vessels where needed.
- Supports kidney damage.
- Increases amount of blood flow to the eye.

Vitamin C is one vitamin that the human body does not produce on its own.

After my intravenous boost, I started taking a very high quality and high-level loose powder via a company called The Allergy Research Group. This was a buffered variety, a very high pure form of ascorbic acid buffered with potassium, calcium and magnesium carbonates. I was severely affected by so many things that I needed this intense boost. Nowadays, I take it, still in loose form from Ancient Purity, it is easily managed and can be adjusted depending on my daily situation. It's also great if you don't like taking tablets.

When combined in a complex variety, I discovered that a collection of B vitamins will support the nervous system, helping with stress and anxiety. This was also one of the first vitamins I would turn to when needing support for my nervous system. I used to take one general multivitamin that incorporated all vitamins and supplements; however, over the years, I have separated out vitamins and minerals and take whatever is required.

One that I didn't take at the time thirty-five years ago but now I include in my ReBalancing Toolkit is vitamin D3 alongside vitamin K2, which ensures the calcium is absorbed easily and reaches the bone mass, while preventing calcified arteries. As many as 60% of the UK population are vitamin D deficient and low levels have been linked to serious health problems in later life.

Vitamin D is a hormone rather than a vitamin; it is required to absorb calcium and phosphate from the gut into the bloodstream and it is mostly produced in the skin in response to sunlight and is also absorbed from food eaten (about 10% of vitamin D is absorbed this way) as part of a healthy balanced diet. It contributes to maintaining normal bones, teeth, muscle function and the normal absorption and utilisation of calcium/phosphorus. Vitamin D3 also plays a part in normal cell division, the immune system's routine function, and healthy inflammatory responses. Vitamin K2 contributes to the maintenance of normal bones and blood coagulation whilst in combination. The major source of our body's vitamin D comes from our own production in the skin. This requires the ultraviolet rays from sunlight to form vitamin D3; the liver and the kidneys are needed to create the active form of vitamin D.

Pause

Supplement ME

Can you consider introducing vitamin C into your life and vitamin D3 + K2?

If you are feeling out of balance, dealing with post-viral fatigue and lethargy, getting over coughs, colds, sinus problems, or generally feeling an immune slump, consider the highest quality of vitamin C you can and make sure it doesn't have any sugar, dairy or yeast in it.

- Ideally, buy it loose as ascorbic acid so you can manipulate how much you need during your days.
- If you're working within a budget, try to get the highest for your budget.
- Seek support and advice from your local independent health food store.

I would encourage you to review the research and data regarding vitamin D3 & K2 as well; as a supplement, the research is now more up to date than ever.

We need a higher dose if we are rebalancing our health.

B: Bye Bye Sugar

As you have read, this was a vast area where I began to see small changes and shifts in my health by going on an anti-candida eating plan. It was the most challenging thing I had to do; it took every ounce of energy I had left to begin to eat in such a different way, however, I saw the beginning of changes in me and a side of Julia that began to return. This was around two years into my ill health and you could say I was grasping at straws and finding different ways of healing, but something inside knew that removing sugar from my life would be transforming.

However, after about four months of eliminating certain foods from my day, I became much worse. I ended up even more lethargic, unable to move, sleeping most of the day, and having more yucky spots and headaches. I was about to give up. I didn't know what was happening to me, but in talking it through with Mum and reading about it further, I knew that what I was experiencing was 'a toxic release'. I was not providing the organisms with the sugar, so they were reducing in number and, in panic, throwing toxicity into my bloodstream. Although this was an awful place to be, I stuck with it; somewhere deep inside me, intuitively, I knew it was all working for my best outcome.

The books that helped me through this were Candida Albicans: Could Yeast Be Your Problem by Leon Chaitow and Candida Albicans by Gill Jacobs; these two books I devoured at the time and I still have to this day.

I was very strict in reducing sugar. Anything that had a relationship to sugar: fructose, glucose, corn syrup, molasses, syrup, honey plus of course I'm including artificial sweetener here, aspartame, a definite no-no. I let go of any fruit for the first nine months, knowing I would allow them back in, but in this early phase, I decided to keep them out.

This entire time was very difficult, it was a new education - every tin, every packet, every jar was scanned and if there was any ounce of sugar in there, it wasn't invited. Life changed for me and also for my family.

Sugar is more prevalent than people think; here are a few examples of products to replace:

- Sweetcorn in a tin.
- Mayonnaise.
- Tomato ketchup.
- Ready-made sauces.
- Bought bread.
- Flavoured crisps.
- Breakfast cereals.
- Alcohol.

Like I have been saying, I was heavily researching – often, I didn't have the energy to do this, so it was slow; I could only do so much on any one day, but I read what I could from the library and sourced resources that were relating to being on an anti-candida diet.

It was hard... no bread, pickles, mature hard cheese, mushrooms, or anything that fermented and became yeasty or sugary.

All of these foods were ultimately feeding the infestation of yeast in my body. Unbeknownst to me after eating, it would feast on it, letting toxins into my bloodstream making me feel incredibly tired, lethargic, bloated and uncoordinated.

I certainly didn't rush into it; I planned when I would start, cleaned up all the foods from the cupboards, and had my alternatives to help begin this new phase.

About six months after those initial four, I began to feel lighter; my brain fog was beginning to lift, my energy levels began to rise, I knew that something was shifting.

I remained eating this way for about fourteen years. I suppose you could say that I wanted to ensure that I wouldn't let the yeast that is usually living peacefully in my colon get out of hand again. This was a bit radical, but as you can understand, I was in charge and had to oversee this change so I could get my life back.

It took a long time before I allowed alcohol back in, and even then, it's rare. We made a lot of food from scratch; again, I couldn't have done this without Mum. My tastebuds loved sugar; I used to seek it out, so the stronghold began to detach once I removed it. I didn't crave it. The only time I struggled was when I was premenstrual and my desire to eat something sweet raised slightly, but I found alternatives such as carob and homemade oat bars, though years later I discovered I had developed an intolerance to oats, most likely caused by the over replacement of oats and the sugars in the carbohydrate.

After about a year, I reintroduced organic honey and fruit but made sure that I ate fresh fruit and not over-ripe fruit (especially bananas when more sugar is produced).

Sugar is the Western diet's downfall – hidden in all our foods, it can have a real detrimental effect on how you feel. It raises our glucose levels and gives us false highs and lows. I'm not suggesting removing it so drastically like I did, unless you have a yeast problem as well, but if you need to rebalance, one of the main things you can do for yourself is remove sugar, even if this is for a few months or so as you apply some other practices that I have shared. Sugar is also a very key component to carbohydrates, so I reduced refined carbs back then.

Pause

You're Sweet Enough

- Do you have a feeling that sugar needs to be removed from your daily life?
- Is it hiding in your store cupboard – look at the tins, jars, bottles, packets, condiments.
- How about your fridge/freezer?
- Think about your cravings... what is on your list?

A huge sign is when you're craving certain foods - this is your body telling you that something is out of whack - our gut reaches out for sugar. Find what you always turn to - it can be a giveaway. You may not have a yeast overgrowth. However, reducing sugar can help hugely with overall feelings of tiredness and sleepy slumps in the afternoons, not forgetting the sugar in alcohol, which can impact in other ways.

B: Probiotic Possibilities

I critically thought through a lot of information; I researched like you wouldn't believe, I did not take anything for granted, I didn't believe just because a health practitioner told me. I had to look for patterns and reviews before knowing what to do. I was looking at the whole picture, not just one tiny chink of it.

When I received all the information sheets from Martin Lev from The ME Action Campaign, I was so interested to read about Candida Albicans and the link with antibiotics, so I asked Dr Griffiths for a list of all the antibiotics I had taken in my life and he very kindly wrote out every single one, including the dates, the actual drug, and the origin of the illness.

I was pretty shocked when I saw, written before me, all the antibiotics I had been on since I was two years old. Forty-three of them up to the age of sixteen. I still have that handwritten list of A5 letter-headed paper. It is mind-boggling to this day.

It was a huge light bulb moment at this acute stage of illness. Although not the exact cause, it was certainly hindering my body's healing capacity. I saw the connection between long term antibiotics and disturbing the gut microbiome, thereby giving candida albicans full control. Candida is an organism that is usually present and stays in balance within the gut. Through many factors such as antibiotics, the pill, steroids, heavy pharmaceutical drugs, poor diet, heightened stress responses, it causes an imbalance in the stomach. It dawned on me that all of the antibiotics had seriously compromised my immune system and when researching it further, I knew that my gut was in a right mess.

That's where probiotics came into the mix, helping to ease and balance my intestinal tract, putting back the good bacteria.

Probiotics will come in many forms. I had a high source of microorganisms such as Lactobacillus acidophilus, Bifidobacterium lactis, Lactobacillus paracasei and Lactobacillus rhamnosus, and because of my intolerances, I made sure that it was in pure form without any additives and no wheat, dairy, soya or egg.

Years ago, I took loose probiotic powder that I made into a drink, which is a great way of taking it as you can also add to smoothies or water. There are many capsules around too. I would always seek independent companies.

> “It feels like I am being poisoned – whenever friends come round to see me, I feel drained, I'm constantly pushing myself, this is no way to live.

Pause

Your Insides Guide

Are your insides telling you something?

- Have you had a history of antibiotics in your life? The pill, steroids, prescription medication?
- Do you suffer from unpredictability with your bowel movements?
- Have you taken probiotics before and given up?
- Do you have bouts of diarrhoea, irritability, intense fatigue, feeling run down after eating, and feeling hugely bloated.
- For any irritability in the gut, seek out Psyllium Husk, which you take before eating.
- A huge area of investigation is the digestive tract and microbiome.

Don't take my word for it, this is about you becoming your own holistic health investigator. Your insides really are your guides.

Our gut is in direct connection with our brain, often we won't be able to sleep based on what is happening in our stomach and vice versa. What further research do you need to do?

B: Echinacea

Echinacea is a North American daisy family plant used in herbal medicine, largely for its antibiotic and wound-healing properties. It is believed that Echinacea is generally taken at the beginning of a cold flu virus; in fact, it can be taken every day throughout the year, it will help to boost a strong foundation of natural immunity. If you then come into contact with viruses, colds, flu, and bugs, your immune system is stronger and better prepared. This again relates to germ theory versus terrain theory.

As mentioned earlier, it's worth repeating, germ theory suggests that germs are what we need to worry about, and we need to keep finding ways to kill them off. Whereas terrain theory argues that if the body is well and balanced, then germs that are a natural part of life and the environment around us will be dealt with by the body without causing sickness.

Antoine Béchamp, the nineteenth-century rival of Louis Pasteur is quoted as saying, "*Germs seek their natural habitat – diseased tissue – rather than being the cause of diseased tissue.*"

Echinacea has been a stable product in my life. Initially, I used a tincture; even with an alcohol base it can be evaporated in warm/hot water, varieties of this particular brand from A. Vogel are where I turn: tablets, tincture and throat spray. If you're pregnant or breastfeeding, as with all remedies and prescriptions, it is usually advised to use your discretion and talk to your midwife/doula doctor or natural health practitioner. Now I always have echinacea throat spray within my bag and by my bedside.

If you're looking for another form of Echinacea, make sure it is produced using extracts of freshly harvested, organically grown echinacea purpurea herb and root, picked fresh and used within twenty-four hours of harvest. The benefit of using freshly harvested herbs has been demonstrated in research - extracts produced from fresh plants contain almost three times more active substances compared with those obtained from equivalent amounts of dried herb.

If you would rather not take a remedy because of the alcohol, you can add it to hot water and let the alcohol evaporate. If you're allergic to the daisy plant, it isn't recommended. I'm seeing quite a number of clients recently who are just succumbing to colds and coughs, generally feeling they're fighting something, tired, yukky and low energy.

Vogel's echinacea throat spray is a must.

Pause

Blooming Daisy

- Would echinacea help strengthen your immune system at the moment?
- What works best for you: tincture, tablets, or throat spray?
- What further investigation do you need to do?
- Do you have any contraindications i.e. are you allergic to the daisy family?

B: Seasonally Organic

When I had to radically eliminate foods from my diet because of the infestation of yeast in my system, I looked at my vegetables' source and quality and I began to rotate vegetables, never relying on one variety for more than a few days.

I began to ask myself - where were they coming from and could I find organic? I knew I wanted to eliminate the chemicals.

Back in the early 90s, supermarkets didn't stock organic vegetables. We discovered through word of mouth that there was an organic farm about fifteen miles away. So off Mum and I trundle. We were amazed by the simple selection. The place was full of vegetables but only a very small variety. We asked the farmer why there was such a small selection and he said it was all related to 'what was in season'.

Of course, this all harks back to the good old days when you bought what was in season: potatoes, carrots, broccoli, sprouts in the winter and radishes, lettuce, peas, beans, corn, strawberries, raspberries in the summer.

We have come to rely on fruit and vegetables all year round from our supermarkets, they have travelled many miles by plane and truck just so we can have strawberries all year round; our countries have different policies about spraying chemicals and unless you're up to scratch with the origins, you never really know where it's coming from. Of course, this isn't how our parents and grandparents used to shop. They would buy, create and store summer fruits to last throughout the year, whether in jams, pickles, or chutneys. Once the freezer became a staple item in many kitchens, fresh fruits could be cooked and frozen, pies could be created.

It was a planner's paradise.

A long time ago, families would plant locally and within their community, in their back gardens. Your soil was your soil. You knew what went into it. The days like this are returning.

I remember when I was about ten, we used to have a man who delivered to each of our streets. His name was Reg, so we called him Reg the Veg. In his brown converted truck, he sold the staple supplies for all households, and I used to help measure out my Mum's order. The day was always exciting when Reg knocked on our door and said, "*I have strawberries today.*" I used to love crunchy carrots and celery to eat, raw peas in the pod when it was their time, and green beans. All of these memories served me well when I had to reorganise my food intake and I began to eat a selection of raw organic vegetables every day. Reg the Veg wasn't organic, but he was seasonal and local from farms nearby.

There wasn't a huge variety in those days, so I would have

whatever was in season, but I'd have it raw, lightly steamed, and organic. My selection did diminish but I knew that what was entering my body had not been sprayed with chemical compounds.

The supermarkets caught up and began to supply a small organic range; this has of course increased over the last twenty-five years and now, although they are more expensive, I make sure that I buy organic produce when I can. Vegetables and fruit are a huge part of my diet and I watch where they come from.

According to the Pesticide Action Network UK, the Dirty Dozen were found to have 210 pesticide chemicals on them. These are: strawberries, spinach, kale, collard/mustard greens, peaches, pears, nectarines, apples, grapes, bell/hot peppers, cherries, blueberries and green beans. This changes yearly so it is always a good idea to check.

The price will be higher for organic products. However, I would rather have a box of selected veg that I use and know is from a good source, than have 'everything' in my fridge and not know where it is from. A great way of sourcing organic is to find your local farm or independent health store, which often has 'organic boxes' from suppliers. You pay a weekly rate and you get delivered a selection of what's in season. Some suppliers may import, if there are organic strawberries available in January from Cuba and you fancy them, then get them. Ideally, let's get growing our fruit and veg again and rekindle this lost skill.

The Clean Fifteen showing the least pesticides are avocados, sweetcorn, pineapple, onions, papaya, frozen peas, aubergine, asparagus, broccoli, cabbage, kiwi, cauliflower, mushrooms, honeydew melon and cantaloupe melon. There is new research from Sally K Norton in her book, called Toxic Superfoods: How Oxalate Overload Is Making You Sick—and How to Get Better, this covers more about the toxins and could be something to explore if you're suffering with inflammation, fatigue, bloating.

Pause

F&V Organically

Look at your vegetable intake and assess what you eat and how you eat it.

- If you look at your plate, what percentage are the vegetables in the meal?
- How much of that vegetable is boiled, roasted, steamed, stir fry?
- Boiled - you're just boiling away any nutrients - steam, quick stir fry, or raw.
- Can you find two organic vegetables and two organic fruit items in your area?
- Where can you buy organic fruit and veg from in your area or nationally? Time for investigation.

If you can, keep it organic and seasonal.

The Second Way

Nourish

to enhance and provide with food or other substances necessary for growth, health and good condition.

There was no particular order to the way I was experimenting, it was dependent on who I was seeing at that time. I used to reflect upon how else could I nourish myself? How could I provide the conditions for my immunity and body to initiate its self-healing capabilities? I knew that this was going to be crucial, don't ask me how I knew at this age.

Back then, I had seen I was eating all of the same grain mostly wheat. Whilst I didn't know much then about carbohydrates and the link to sugars, I recognised that perhaps there was a trigger. If I fast forward to the present day I find when I eat less grain, the less bloated I feel. However back then, I removed the majority of the main grains that would give my digestion a rest. There is a great deal now around eating low carbohydrates as well as intermittent fasting so you may find you experiment with this whole area, seek advice from a practitioner.

Remember this is about small manageable changes and steps to feeling lighter and less fatigued. What grains are you eating the most of is often the first place to look and reducing refined carbohydrate intake.

I took it back to the very basics and started with grains.

From what information was available to me then, I decided that releasing and rotating grains was a good place to start, as well as not mixing protein, fats and carbs in one meal. I began to look at water and the source, exploring how hydrated I was and the quality of that hydration. Then I turned to clearing out any unnecessary chemicals that I was using in the home. I intuitively went barefoot outside, I didn't know the implications of that but later discovered the huge benefits, and I turned to journalling as a way of nourishing myself and conversing with my inner Julia.

N: Food Combining

After I discovered I had severe candidiasis - an infestation of yeast in my system that was diminishing my immunity - I had to embrace a new eating schedule, removing key foods and toxins from my diet, and boy, my life took on a completely different regime. It was here I began to learn a very important lesson - rotate and release the grain.

I recognised that I had come to rely on wheat as my primary carbohydrate source, eating far too much of it for breakfast, lunch and dinner. Bread, pasta and flour, this isn't just me, it is predominantly the Western diet. Wheat flour is used in all manner of condiments and added as a filler within so many recipes. Wheat is also heavily chemically sprayed with glyphosate, a herbicide applied to the leaves of plants to kill both broadleaf plants and grasses with much controversy, this is in the UK and internationally. Therefore, you're not just dealing with wheat as a grain but the chemical composition of this grain, which has changed over the centuries. If we milled our own wheat, the nutrients would still be present, now with industrial production, there is rarely anything left, which is why fortified vitamins are added back in, being synthetic, they too often cause a problem. Ancient grains for example, einkorn, emmer, khorasan/kamut, durum and spelt refers to heritage grains pre-hybridisation of the modern wheat, if ground by hand they may be tolerated better. At the time, it was very rare so I didn't have the opportunity to try it.

I began to release the main grains to give my digestion a break.

After letting go of wheat, I began to introduce rye and short grain brown rice. However, what I did discover was the food combining system of not mixing proteins and carbohydrates in the same meal. This was known back then as The Hay Diet and it helped to show me how to separate out these groups to allow better digestion and initiate balance. It really meant cooking from scratch where possible and staying very simple. A few years into my eating, new pastas began emerging using different flours and legumes, these were still incredibly starchy, so although I tried them, I found it spiked my tiredness and bloating.

I began to replace oats in my diet, but fast forward many years, I can't tolerate oats because I overcompensated for them. I just replaced oats for the wheat. Oat milk is a definite no-no because it causes bloating, if you're drinking oat milk and feeling lethargy, bloating or brain fog, release from your diet for a week to see if your symptoms decrease.

I became very astute to what triggered reactions within myself. I would note down how I felt physically and emotionally because, as we now know, our gut is deeply connected to our brain and the link between the two is deep. If this resonates with you the gut microbiome needs more investigation.

For now, it's about recognising that food is really our medicine as Hippocrates stated. *"Let Food Be Thy Medicine and Medicine Be Thy Food."*

Years later I came to see how refined carbohydrates can contribute to many health issues. There is much discussion around eating keto/low carb/animal based/vegetarian/vegan suffice to say my aim here is to encourage you to explore this Way of not mixing carbs and protein in one meal, rotate or release grains, give your digestion a rest from the one grain you eat the most.

Explore your nutrition. Cook from scratch and develop meals yourself, know from the outset what is in your food, research and investigate proteins, carbohydrates and fats.

Pause

Release the Grain

Take a look at how you eat in your daily practice.

- Do you rely upon one grain? Which one, wheat, rice, oats?
- Start to look at how you can release this grain and assess how you feel.
- Can you keep your protein meals separate from carbohydrate meals?
- Do you need to clear out your store cupboard?
- Begin to investigate, research and read up on low carb, no carb, food combining, carnivore.

Note: This will be very different if you are coeliac or have known allergies.

N: Hydration

I discovered very early on that drinking water straight from the tap wasn't good because of the chemicals that were added to the water e.g., usually either chlorine or chloramine which kills disease-causing germs such as Salmonella, Campylobacter, and norovirus in addition to fluoride which is added - each local authority will have the source of how much fluoride they add. Fluoride is a chemical that does need to be investigated as there are serious implications. When I was trying to take all pressures and stressors off my immune system, my water source was crucial and another factor to consider.

We are 70% water by volume. Yet molecularly, we are 99.95% water molecules.

I discovered that the brain and heart are composed of 73% water. The lungs are about 83% water. The skin contains 64% water, muscles and kidneys are 79%, and even the bones are watery: 31%. As Isabel Friend, Water Ambassador says, "*We are water beings as much as we are human beings.*"

Back in the 90s, we bought a standard water filter which

was new in the day; this was the first step for us as a family. Fast forward to the present day, I have a water distiller that removes most contaminants, such as chlorine, fluoride, graphene oxide, heavy metals and parasites. I then restructure the water with salts and energise it. I have a copper carafe that I use for helping to remove toxins out the water. I am beginning to truly immerse myself in the real essence of water. For now, for you, it's about exploring what you drink, how you drink it and when.

In the 90s, I was interviewed for an article about my illness for my local newspaper. Consequently, a woman contacted me about using crystals in my water - in fact, she sent me three garnet crystals that I was to place in my water filter. I wasn't sure at the time what benefit this would give me; I was twenty-two and I would try anything. I was investigating and this was my test.

What I knew for sure was that I had to drink the best possible water for me – a good source of it, to help recharge my mitochondria (the powerhouse and energy batteries in our cells) and make a concerted effort to drink. If you drink water from plastic water bottles don't leave them in your car, they can then overheat and the plastic can begin to break down components into the water that is then drunk.

About five years after healing, I came across a book called The True Power of Water by Dr Masaru Emoto. This book asked me to consider the characteristics of water and contemplate how water could improve my health and life. It went into great detail based on his experiments that showed water could change its molecular composition. His research confirmed that sending gratitude to water improves its molecular structure and deteriorates when it is polluted. This was discovered by freezing the water and taking photographs of the water droplets after being exposed to blessings and loving statements as well as polluted water and negative statements. This was the beginning of my journey into the realm of consciousness, and I began to see how we are so interconnected with each other and nature around us.

If you have seen the film What The Bleep you will recognise this, as within the film, the actress started drawing love hearts all over her body to send love to herself. As she knew that water within her would respond.

Only in this year of book writing and researching, I discovered two inspirational women. Veda Austin, a water researcher, dedicating the last ten years to observing and photographing the life of water. She believes that water is fluid intelligence, observing itself through every living organism. Her primary area of focus is photographing water in its 'state of creation', the space between liquid and ice. She produces remarkable crystallographic photos where water reveals its awareness of creation and thought and intention through imagery. The other is Isabel Friend, international ambassador of water, public speaker and educator, seamlessly blending science and spirit into a comprehensive cosmology of water wisdom. She provides practical insights of health, hydration and biology. Because as she says "*Water is life, and life is sacred*."

Somewhere within my investigation, even back then in the 90s. I knew that water was key.

Pause

Water In, Water Out

Reflect on your water source.

- Where is the best place for you to get your water from?
- Can you invest in a water filter? What type suits?
- What about your shower and washing your body.
- Notice how much water you really drink.
- Begin to incorporate more hydration into your daily life - this could be from watermelon.
- Investigate hydrogen water.

Start blessing your water; what I do is I print off pieces of printed labels that say things like 'I love you', or 'Thank You, 'I am grateful for you', 'I feel blessed having you'. Then I stick them with the words facing the water on my bottle. I will wrap my hands around the glass and express something inwardly to the water. I also have a blue glass bottle that I will fill with water and energise via the sun outside for an hour or so.

Dr Masaru Emoto's book is such an interesting read, here you will see that the molecules change when we are kind to water.

Veda Austin Crystallographer, takes this one step further

around her own freezing technique showing how we can communicate with water ourselves at home.

Isabel Friend will also open another door of water hacking and you will be transformed into a dynamic new portal.

N: Chemical Clear Out

Smell had a huge impact on my sensory system. What exactly was I inhaling, using and more so, what was I putting on my body, or immersing myself in? I began to look at what chemical products my body was absorbing through my skin. As I researched chemicals more and more, I was becoming more conscious of the ingredients of the products and the manufacturer. This then led me to consider all the artificial fake smells around me. Things that I thought were in my control but, in fact, I didn't know what was in them. I began to switch basic products. This didn't happen all at once, but slowly and gradually I found more products that suited me and were still working.

Around this time, the term GMO began to surface - genetically modified organism, which meant changing an organism's genes in a laboratory setting. Manufacturers of GMO products want to improve the product or gain a commercial advantage; this may include food items, or grains for agriculture. There are no long-term studies relating to the impact on human health and the interference of genetically changing the structure, so long-term effects are not known. I intuitively felt that this was not the way I wanted to go. There are no such things as 'seedless grapes', Quorn is a lab-made product, and now we are in the Frankenstein territory of lab-grown artificial meat.

My Mum's close Australian cousins sent me a book called Toxic Chemical Free Living and Recovery from ME/CFS by Trixie Whitmore. This book was an eye-opener for me and it profiled Trixie's story of healing from ME and how she discovered she was intolerant to the chemicals in her environment. Consequently, this was another layer in my restoration to stop using anything artificial and chemically prepared, either topically or via inhalation as I knew they were being absorbed into my whole-body system.

The veil was lifting; I began to see sunscreen protection filled with chemicals - seemingly, this was the opposite of what it was trying to do - knowing about how the skin absorbs whatever is placed upon it, I didn't want synthetics on my skin so I would seek out sun protection with naturally based sunscreens.

Chemicals coated onto shoes can produce an intolerant reaction, new carpet, wood glue, preservatives and paint to name but a few. Any new chemical smells and perfumes can irritate your body and nervous systems, so bear this in mind when you're assessing. It was about this time that I also stopped using products that were tested on animals. This felt out of sync with what I was trying to achieve and that was a total removal of stressors on my body, mind and spirit. I began here.

I started with the following:

- Furniture polish - stopped using pronto.
- Fly spray - never again.
- Deodorisers/room sprays - avoided commercially synthetic sprays. Made own with water, essential oils.

Then, I moved on to these:

- Under arm deodorants – stuck to natural deodorant and not antiperspirant.
- Toothpaste, homeopathic, herbal, mineral - without fluoride or synthetic chemicals.
- Washing powder/liquid - sourced one that was for sensitive skin. Unprocessed as possible, less chemical.
- Perfume/aftershave - natural perfumes based on essential oils.
- Shampoo – excluded sodium lauryl sulphate, parabens.
- Shower gel - using bars of natural organic soap.
- Cleanser, toner, moisturiser - replaced with organic coconut oil, rose water, sweet almond oil, rosehip, or carrot oil. Started to make my own.
- Cleaning products - the less chemical the better/sourced, vegan based, not tested on animals. I began to make my own with vinegar and essential oils, bicarbonate of soda and lemons.

Pause

The Chemical Bothers

There is so much more to this particular topic of chemicals on our skin, in our homes, in our environment, but notice what is irritating you right now.

- What are you using?
- Can you make a fundamental switch? Basic switches could be from the list above, items that are in your control. All these can assist with nourishing your body system and taking stressors off.
- What is around you? E.g., cleaning products
- Do you work in an environment that uses chemicals? Could they be impacting you?

The Chemical Bothers are asking you to notice what is bothering you.

N: Earthing

When my head felt all over the place and my spirit felt shaky, I would go outside, take my shoes and socks off and let my bare feet feel the earth, the grass and the soil. When I could barely lift my head up from my pillow and getting dressed was a real chore, I would hold some soil in my hands.

This is called Earthing, sometimes referred to as Grounding.

I didn't know about the term Earthing back in the 90s, but I somehow felt the benefit of bare feet/hands connecting to grass, earth and soil (even concrete, just not tarmac). Even when the weather was pretty rotten, I would do this – just a few steps for bare feet or hands to reach the earth. Many years later, when I read the book *Earthing by Clinton Ober, Stephen Sinatra, Martin Zucker,* I realised what I was doing was from a very intuitive place.

Grounding, or Earthing, refers to connecting with the earth plane.

This is heavily researched.

Because of our modern rubber/plastic soled shoes and our exposure to technology around us, we don't have this natural electrical connection to the earth unless walking barefoot.

Why do we need to?

According to *Earthing*:

"*The Earth is a massive reservoir of negatively charged free electrons. Without a connection to this reservoir, the cells in our body are unable to balance the positive charge.*"

Our modern environment is full of a wide spectrum of electromagnetic radiation, from computers, mobile phones and masts, radio and TV broadcasts, WIFI, Bluetooth, power lines, domestic wiring, and other electrical appliances. This electromagnetic radiation induces voltages in our bodies, disrupting the trillions of subtle electrical communications, which are a vital part of the function of our body's systems.

On a less tangible level, it may also be that the connection we make with the earth actually carries information and helps align us with the greater network of intelligence of our plane.

We know this, don't we? Can you feel it when you're barefoot and out in the grass? How can connecting to the earth element help you?

- Improved immune function.
- Improved digestion
- Improved sleep.
- Rapid healing of injuries.
- Improved blood circulation.
- Harmonisation and stabilisation of the body's basic biological rhythms.
- Accelerated recovery from intense athletic activity.

- Reduction of inflammation.
- Reduced stress / anxiety / irritability.
- Reduced electro sensitivity.

You know that feeling, when you're on holiday and you have walked barefoot on the beach, your feet in the sand, toes immersed in the sea, or legs dangling in a gorgeous running stream, you return feeling centred, recharged and energised.

We often think that this is because of the holiday itself (which, of course, is a factor) but when you look at the scientific proof, it is because we have earthed ourselves.

Now, there are many grounding mats and sheets that create an earth source for you when you're sleeping or working from a computer. A few years ago, I bought a grounding computer pad, which I use when I'm working with my laptop, plus a grounding sheet to add to the bottom of my bed.

Pause

Ground Yourself

A very simple, straightforward thing is to find the earth and step on it.

Finding a way to connect and recalibrate through the earth is nourishing and in combination with other prompts, this will help you earth your body system.

- How often do you go barefoot and outside to have contact with the earth?
- If you can't, can you immerse your hands in the soil?
- Would you consider a grounding mat for night or by your computer?

N: Journalling

I turned to keeping a journal in the first year of being ill. I had always kept a diary, but this was different.

I was writing my heart out.

There was no method to my journalling. I wrote about my day, what was happening, how I felt, which appointment I had that day, and what I wanted to do next.

Not every day was completed, there were many days that I just was not well enough to hold a pen. However, I did have it by my bedside and it became a focus for writing my insides out.

Journalling helped me. It still does to this day.

The time to sit with my journal and my pen was sacred.

Writing with a pen always connected me to my inner world, it nourished me. Now, when I type on a laptop, I am usually writing from excerpts that I have taken from my journal.

My journal time was very important to me, I created a practise around it and I allowed my inner emotions and spirit self to be heard.

- I turned to my journal when I felt out of sorts, upset, despondent, sad.
- I turned to my journal if I felt angry and needed to explore my inner world.
- I turned to my journal if I felt lost or mixed up about decisions.
- I turned to my journal to explore ideas about my future.
- I turned to my journal when I felt my health was shifting and I was happy.
- I spent those early years tucked up inside my journals and I still have them to this day. When I look back and read them, my eyes glaze over as I read the heart of a twenty-one year old who was doing her utmost to find her way out of the maze.
- There is no right or wrong way of starting this.

In my current journal practice, I make sure I have a journal that makes me smile every time I open it. My journal was another version of therapy. It helped me to process all that was happening. Often, I would come home and write about the therapy session and what insights I had. To this day I turn to my journal to write.

I had to talk to someone else who could help me see what was happening to me, allowing me to talk, with no judgement or preconceived notions of my life.

My journal was one part of that relationship.

> “Listen to your inner voice, Jules, it will give you the answers.

Pause

Write Your Inside Out

Find the Journal, one you will enjoy opening; bright, patterned, plain, lined, it's what you gravitate towards.

What's on the cover to inspire you?

Choose your pen. This is crucial! A lovely flowing pen is required when writing in a journal, something that glides along the page.

Choose a certain time that you'll set aside which is good for you to sit and write. Fifteen minutes is a lovely way to begin.

Create a routine.

Let me give you some prompts to get you started:

- What's on your mind right in this very moment, reading this?
- What is causing you the most discomfort?
- What stands out the most?

The third Way

Support

a source of comfort, assistance, or encouragement

I turned to what is often referred to as complementary and alternative approaches (although I refer to them as original and natural) because this was where I could see the most support for what was happening with me. From the beginning of seeking out homeopathy, I found my way to discovering reflexology, aromatherapy, Bach flower remedies, counselling and reiki. There were many that I tried that I haven't included in here, those I have included impacted me deeply in combination with each other and everything else I was doing.

The key for me was to stay open, fully engage in the treatments, asking questions from the practitioner whilst learning from their knowledge and experience.

S: Aromatherapy

Something quite momentous happened in 1991. Sue Bell, a hypnotherapist I was seeing said, *"I feel you'd really benefit from going to see Maria Barrington, she's an aromatherapist and reflexologist."*

This referral shifted me onto another timeline.

Maria was instrumental in helping me change the trajectory and added a whole new dimension to my future well-being. A wonderful holistic therapist, reflexologist, aromatherapist and reiki master who, thankfully, I still have in my life today, thirty six years later.

We embarked on a journey together. She didn't know anything about ME, nor the intense muscle pain or flu-like symptoms that I had. When I first met Maria, she suggested the first couple of treatments would be aromatherapy massages. We both thought that this was going to deeply relax my muscles and prepare them for healing. What we didn't know and would never have guessed was how exhausting they would be for me.

She knew that having a high quality essential oil diluted in a sweet almond carrier oil would be absorbed into my system and that was the good bit, however the intense massage therapy was totally exhausting me. Pressure points on the back of legs, front, arms, midriff, neck, shoulders; it was absolutely beautiful. However, after that first session, I slept constantly for most of two days. Some may say this was a good thing and in hindsight, it may have been, but I didn't want to feel this intense exhaustion again at that time. So she decided to focus on reflexology, continuing to use specific essential oils that would help my body system on my feet.

The three oils that stood out for me that she used a lot were geranium, clary sage and rose. These three have now been my staple supply for the past thirty years, I turn to them to add into my bath, (six to eight drops in total), or to add to massage oil for my feet, or placed in water, or on a tissue by my bed.

Clary sage is a wonderful essential oil, which is often used for depression (to me it smells like chocolate!) Its greatest benefit lies in its calming and sedating influence on the nerves, emotions, female functions, kidneys and digestive system. It also helps with skin conditions like acne, boils, ulcers and cools painful muscles and joints.

Geranium is related to hormones and is an oil that helps to balance, steadying the mind and emotions, while stimulating the adrenal cortex and balancing the hormonal system, stimulating the lymphatic system.

Rose (Otto), this oil is pure love, healing the heart, especially during times of grief. It not only fights depression, grief, anger and fear, but also looks after your heart and digestive system while being the most wonderful remedy for female problems and one of the best oils to use on the skin.

As time passed, I would always be mindful of any oil that I

diffused when it came to the animals in my home, so always check what you're diffusing and don't do it next to animal beds or confined spaces. I don't tend to use electric aromatherapy distillers. I prefer the ones with a night light underneath, this way I can control the output.

Pause

Essential Smells

Dig deeper into essential oils, seek out the different benefits; choose one and absorb in its properties, either via a bath, a diffuser or a massage. You may find that a massage may really suit you today. Now I delight in a massage, where I go to balance. I read somewhere that massage is the new psychotherapy as it releases stored memory from our cells.

Alternatively, smells can also irritate.

- Do you know what smells irritate you? These are often what need to be released in your living space of organisation.
- Find exceptional quality for your oils - organically grown without chemical spray is better.
- It is advised that essential oils are only used after a woman's first trimester of pregnancy.

S: Reflexology

I feel reflexology is undervalued for those that haven't experienced it so intensely like I have.

It is certainly not new. The art of reflexology can be traced back over two thousand years to ancient Egypt, India, and China. Reflexology as we know it today is attributed to the work of Eunice Ingham, an American therapist. Eunice mapped out reflex points on the feet and hands that corresponded to all of the organs, glands and parts of the body. Her original work is taught exclusively by the school she founded, The International Institute of Reflexology.

As Maria told me, the ancient therapy of reflexology could help to balance my immune system and at the same time balance my mind as well as energetically work with my body system, which was very much struggling at that time.

In those early days, when visiting Maria for treatment, I would cry out in pain as she moved gently across another zone.

"*What's that*?" I'd quietly ask.

"*That's your colon*," she'd reply, "*it's very congested*."

I went weekly for several years; I saved what little money I had coming in and put it towards this treatment. Somewhere deep inside of me, I know that it greatly impacted my total body, mind and spirit.

In the early days of ill health, Mum used to do her style of foot massage for me. I'd lie in bed; she'd bring a chair to the end of the bed and pull back the quilt revealing my feet. She placed them on another pillow and spent another thirty minutes gently kneading and massaging them. After a while, we realised what hurt and what didn't and with applying pressure, you move through the pain. We would have a map of the feet there so she could see what was niggling.

Often, I get asked what was 'it' that helped me to get better and I always say it was a combination of approaches. However, reflexology with Maria was a very important component; her emerging knowledge in how to support my whole body, mind and spirit made a huge difference to my health. As a gentle tool for healing, I still turn to it to balance my whole body system today.

Pause

Feet Know

There are times when we just don't give our feet any attention. If you can experience a reflexology treatment and you know of a reputable and qualified therapist, I would encourage you to go and make this part of your journey. Any form of attention on our feet will also impact balancing our parasympathetic nervous system and subsequently, our body.

You can do this with a buddy, your husband, wife, daughter, sister, and then go for it. Experience this feeling of applying pressure to the points on the feet.

The map of the feet is also reflected in the hands, tongue, eye, and ear.

If you have visited a Traditional Chinese Medicine practitioner, or acupuncturist, you will find that your eye will be examined as well as your tongue, and ears too.

You therefore can give yourself a treatment on your hands. However, having someone do this for you adds to the healing. If you haven't experienced reflexology, see if it resonates with you and your back to health journey.

S: Bach Flower Remedies

Back in the early 90s, I discovered Bach flower remedies. I felt a very deep need to discover as much as possible about using flowers to help my emotions. I can't recall how I stumbled upon them, most likely a health food shop, an article in a magazine or the library. I devoured *The Healer Within by Dr Edward Bach*, because I felt so unwell, my emotions were taking a beating, so I thought there could be something for me to explore. Here I was, back living at home with my parents, having left two years earlier to set up a new life, working and earning. Having had a taste of independence, now I was back in the fold, totally and completely dependent. I was walking with a stick and felt like the illness had 'broken me'.

“ Breathe deeply, I write.

Bach flower remedies are a safe and natural method of healing discovered by Dr Edward Bach from 1920 – 1930s in England. They gently restore the balance between mind and body by casting out negative emotions such as fear, worry, hatred and indecision, which interfere with the equilibrium. The remedies allow peace and happiness to return so that the body is free to heal itself. Made from wildflowers they are safe for the whole family including children, animals, pets, plants etc, and are preserved in brandy and are gluten free.

At the time, being in brandy wasn't something that bothered me, even with the yeast overgrowth; I knew I needed to explore what worked for me, though I soon learnt I could evaporate the alcohol in warm water.

I devoured his book and decided to self-select and felt pulled to take gentian, olive and wild oat.

Gentian, according to Dr Bach, '*is for those who are easily discouraged, they are progressing well in illness and in daily life, but any small delay causes doubt and soon disheartens them*'. Yes, that sounded like me. I was trying so hard to move through this and not give up, but felt I had knock backs all the time.

Dr Bach explained that olive could be helpful for '*those who have suffered much mentally or physically and are so exhausted and weary that they feel they have no more strength to make any effort. Daily life is hard work for them, without pleasure*'. I knew this would assist gentian.

Wild oat was for '*those who have ambitions to do something of prominence in life, who wish to have much experience, and to enjoy all that is possible for them, to take life to the full. Their difficulty is to determine what occupation to follow; as although their ambitions are strong, they have no calling which appeals to them above all others. This may cause delay and dissatisfaction*'. I was in a complete crossroads career wise because everything had come to a standstill.

I had many physical symptoms related to muscle spasms,

flu-like shivers, colds, headaches, sore throat, back pain, muscle weakness, lack of coordination and brain fog. However, I did feel that these remedies were helping my emotional self - somewhere, deep inside me, I was helping myself to do something, to shift something. Even though it wasn't translating into the physical body.

I also used Rescue Remedy, which is a preparation featuring five original remedies used in emergencies and accidents, e.g., sudden shock, exams, presentations, interviews. Any situation where anxiety was heightened. I found this original essence to be so valuable for me when I had to approach a particular situation or meeting, maybe a consultation where I had to explain my health timeline. This would often leave me feeling drained but also the build-up to the meeting, or seeing a new practitioner would do the same thing. The five flower essences included are as follows:

- Rock Rose: positive potential is courage and presence of mind.
- Impatiens: positive potential is less hastiness in thought and action.
- Clematis: positive potential is a lively interest in the world around you.
- Star of Bethlehem: positive potential is being strong.
- Cherry Plum: positive potential is serenity with the ability to think and act rationally.

The wonderful thing about Rescue Remedy is that it also came in a cream format, which was very helpful for me when my spots were exploding. It also helped with bangs, bruises, knocks, and actual cuts, especially a paper cut! I wouldn't put it on an open wound; however, once the skin was beginning to heal, I would use a thin layer to help the self-healing capacity of my body system. With my three young nieces at the time, we used to call it 'magic cream' as it was also in a bright yellow tube, they would also ask for this magic cream if they had hurt themselves.

Bach flower remedies can be integrated with other holistic approaches as well as conventional Western medicine, I went on to study Level 1 and Level 2 Bach flower remedies with The Bach Centre, in Oxfordshire - such a wonderful addition to our ReBalancing Toolkit.

Pause

Get Bach

With thirty eight flowers in the system, you may wonder how to go about choosing the right remedy. Bach Remedies created 'The Remedy Chooser'.

Divided into the seven emotional categories as determined by Dr Bach, each section works by asking you some simple questions, which should help determine which remedies you need.

Visit www.bachremedies.com, you will find a button to click to 'choose the Bach essence for you.'

Following the prompts, you will begin to see what flower essences may be helpful for you right now. It is always important to select what really 'feels' rather than what you 'think'.

Go with your gut instinct.

Every. Time.

S: Counselling

When it had been confirmed that I had ME, I knew I needed to talk about my situation. I was so weak and struggling daily, I felt that I was a hindrance to Mum and Dad, Mum in particular, who was doing her best to be optimistic and I know that she was crying to herself away from me - something we discussed many years later in our reflections of this time. I knew I needed to talk to someone who was independent of her, so I didn't have to burden her with the inner wobbles of my mind. I was nearly twenty-two, feeling that life already was playing awful tricks on me. I contacted the British Association of Counselling, now called BACP. (British Association for Counselling and Psychotherapy) to find a practitioner in my area. I was still not working so finding somewhere where I could cover the cost was crucial.

I was so fortunate to discover COMPASS, a charity based in Liverpool that had volunteer counsellors with a donation envelope at the end of the session. This proved to be a lifeline for me. Mum would drop me off, wait for me for sixty minutes or do a little bit of shopping, though that time wouldn't give her long, and then she would return. She asked me if it went well but didn't intrude or prod. I too, kept the sessions to myself. They provided me with an independent space to cry, be upset, explore, be angry, and reflect upon everything happening to me in a genuine, empathic, non-judgemental environment. This inspired me a few years later to train as a counsellor as I saw great value in this profession.

Throughout those years of ill health, I turned to counselling for different situations to help me deal with the feelings and emotions of being ill for a long time and the consequences of that. I gained weight due to inactivity and this upset me so much. I sought out another counsellor for this who helped with my body image, and in later years I went to see different counsellors who had experience in certain areas that I felt could help me process what I was going through.

There was never any time when I didn't see counselling as a positive addition to my healing journey, it gave me independent space to hear myself speak out loud to someone who was not connected. This would usually be all person-centred counselling where I found that the sessions always unravelled at my own pace, nothing was ever forced or directed, we used creativity sometimes to enhance the sessions, which really appealed to me and gave my illness and innermost thoughts another voice. From a very young age, I recognised that talking independently in a counselling setting was helpful and a strength to reach out, not a weakness. It therefore felt a natural progression and a complete career change to begin training as a counsellor so that I could be a professional, independent support for others.

In the early days, Dr Griffiths talked of antidepressants, but

I just didn't understand why I would take them when I was not dealing with a depressive illness but the fallout of feelings of being ill for a long time. It felt like it would have consequences and I didn't want to add another consequence to the mix of long-term antibiotics that were playing out in my current health situation. It was here though that I began to research into antidepressants and what they were in fact doing to the body system and what side effects they would bring.

> “Strong and heavy feelings have been my constant companion for weeks. I am trying hard to regain some good health and a life again.

Pause

Voice It

It is a strength to reach out to speak to an independent counsellor, not a weakness, whether in a professional or communal situation. Finding that individual who you can turn to process and explore what is going on in your life, is extremely healing. I feel that people are anxious about digging up the past and reliving any trauma; when this is managed carefully, considerately and compassionately, you may find that you don't relive or dig up. Counselling does need to always move at your pace and you are in the driving seat.

If you're struggling currently with your health, or the health of a loved one, perhaps caring for a family member, or there is something troubling you with your relationships, work, children or home life, reach out to someone and find support.

What is coming up for you here?

S: Reiki

Reiki is a Japanese form of energy medicine where reiki practitioners use their hands to connect to the vital life force energy all around, this being transferred through the palms of the practitioner to the client in order to encourage the body's innate capacity to self-heal. Rei means 'universal' and ki translates as 'energy'.

A friend mentioned a reiki practitioner she had visited; I had been experiencing some shifts and movements with my health and was beginning to see that I was moving in the right direction, therefore, I was very open to receiving different types of intervention especially between the mind, body and spirit.

Back then I didn't know really what the session would be like, I had no idea what was really happening but I had a strong feeling that this would be a good thing to do.

I was not wrong.

As I lay there on the massage couch, I felt deep relaxation flooding into me, and a peaceful feeling within me that 'all was well and would be well'. I felt tingling and heat; in further treatments, I felt cold and saw vibrant colours before my eyes. However, after the first couple of sessions, it seemed I had some sort of relapse. I slept even more than I had before, though my flu-like symptoms flared up.

I really didn't know what was going on.

Was this a good thing for me?

It was talking to my practitioner who told me that I was probably experiencing a 'healing crisis'. This sometimes happens when shifts are taking place, it was nothing to be worried about.

This too shall pass.

I stuck with it and experienced more and more relaxation. I was discovering more about the world of energy, electrical and magnetic - the elements that nourish and maintain all living things. The Field around us that we can all connect to when we sit in stillness. When these energies flow uninterrupted, there is balance, harmony and ease within, around us, and we experience a sense of well-being. There is dis-ease, dis-order, and chaos when energy is disrupted, interrupted, interfered with and congested.

My body was yearning for harmony, well-being, energy and vitality.

When we have many stressors on our body, mind and spirit we have to turn to ways to unblock and remove them.

So, embarking on a course of reiki sessions I knew this was going to help me to balance - to find my centre once again.

In essence reiki treatments can help the body physically, emotionally and spiritually, being a tradition that is open to any belief system.

Again, I knew this wasn't the total answer for me but it was a way that I wanted to include.

It wasn't long for me to get pulled into the field of reiki after this first treatment and 5 years after I became well, I took my first attunement with Maria, who had subsequently become a Reiki Master. I gently spent the next few years doing my level 2 and Reiki Master level and I use this in my day-to-day life for myself, for clients, and for animals.

When I'm out of balance – it is often because I am not self-healing on a regular basis.

'As running water smooths the jagged edges of a rock until it is small enough to roll away, Reiki flows to the areas of need, soothing and supporting the body's natural ability to heal itself.'

Usui Shiki Ryoho

Pause

Radiant Energy

Some of you may be familiar with reiki, perhaps you are attuned or are thinking about having a session. For others, this may be very new.

Some questions to ask yourself:

- Are you giving your energy away to others?
- If you're attuned, are you giving yourself a daily self-healing?
- If this is new to you, do you wish to include this in your research?
- Where can you go for treatment?

When you read these questions, reflect upon how you feel reiki may support you.

The fourth Way

Cocoon

to envelop in a protective or comforting way.

I found myself naturally cocooning. It wasn't something I planned; it happened organically because I was building these different approaches into my day. You could say I was weaving my own cocoon. Only when I began to write this book and look back at how I was restoring my health did I recognise what this meant for me. Cocoon was a way to protect myself and my boundaries, whether it was ditching the news, learning the art of being still in P&Q (peace and quiet), saying no, creating a screen around sleep as well as learning about technology and EMF's (electromagnetic frequencies) in later years all of this enabled me to cocoon and I realised just how important this was for me.

Unstable and shaky boundaries are a huge area that deplete our energy, so identifying ways to not only cocoon but also protect ourselves and our environment is crucial when we are restoring our health and vitality.

Co: Ditch the News

In the early days of seeing Maria for reflexology, she handed me a book at the end of a session, it was called You Can Heal Your Life by Louise Hay.

"*Here, have this,*" she said, "*I haven't got time to read it.*"

To say I devoured this book is an understatement. It made a huge impact on me at the time and became a firm friend; if you saw it now, you would realise how fond I was as the pages are falling out. There are many gems to glean from this book, but one of them that I began to integrate into my daily life was removing the constant drip feed of negative influences from my life.

What do I mean by that?

Louise Hay suggested to stop watching the news late at night.

That's just what I did. I used to watch the news at 10 p.m. and decided to take it one step further and I stopped watching the news throughout the day. I also didn't listen to the news every hour on the radio; you would find me turning off two minutes before the hour and turning back on two minutes after. This was before the rise of the Internet and multi-cable channels, so I wasn't even bombarded with it like we are now.

My intention here was to cleanse my environment. This was related to the energetic outpouring of such negativity that I didn't want late at night before bed. Show me The Good News channel and I'll be there.

This was the beginning of what I would later on call Cocoon.

I would avoid any negative drama or documentary and I certainly wasn't the kind of person that enjoyed watching horror or violent films, they just weren't on my radio wave. I didn't listen to songs with lyrics that were low and dense.

I found that as I planned my way to bed, I surrounded myself with different practices that would not tell me who had died suddenly, who'd been murdered, what conflict was maiming people, who and what I 'should' fear in society and the world around me. Of course, I was still abreast of what was happening, but I didn't drip feed 'news' into my subconscious mind.

'Drip feed' being two very important words here.

Negative drip feed from news, media, films, and radio has a big impact on you, creating a fear mindset that turns on your inner alarm, causing hormone disruption in your body and mind. Reducing this, I found, took an extra stressor off my body, mind and spirit.

This is where I began to assess the differences between when I was absorbing positive energy and when I wasn't. It was where I used my sixth sense, becoming quiet. I would ask myself – 'does this feel right to watch and listen to?'

The intention was for me to release all that wasn't supporting my healing environment; that also meant people that were draining me.

Over the years, I have added to this a great deal. Now I don't have live TV and I'm very selective about what I watch. I am mindful about mainstream media. Back in the day I would follow a series but you had to wait for the next episode, there was no on demand or instant access. We're talking Around the World in 80 Days with Michael Palin, Roseanne, The Golden Girls, Poirot, Neighbours, and who remembers Hitman and Her? This gave me the illusion of being out clubbing on a Saturday night, whilst I was awake in the early hours of the morning ill in bed. There are benefits of television, particularly films, as you'll see in the Fifth Way, Create, sometimes a good way to relax and switch off, however if dealing with ongoing health problem, it can often be even more draining, watching external negative drama, so seeking a relaxing pursuit to move through the evening to bed can really soothe your nervous system. Adverts and high dopamine rushes, the stimulus of colour and LED lighting can intensify symptoms. With regards to the news on tv and radio, be consciously aware that it is a constant drip feed.

Step away and watch the theatre unfold.

Pause

Release the Drip

Take some time to note how much media you watch and how it makes you feel. What can you do to release this negative drip?

- Do you have the radio and news channels on in the background, drip-feeding into your subconscious?
- Do you really want to avoid programmes on TV but your partner, parent, husband, wife, son/daughter watches and you feel discomfort from it?
- Can you take a break from news channels late at night? Experiment with that.
- What are you consuming with technology that is possibly evoking a fear narrative within you? e.g. films, documentaries, video games; do you feel sad, upset, wounded by the time it has all finished?
- Are there family, friends, or colleagues who drain you on the phone or in real time? There is also a release that has to happen here too.

Co: Peace & Quiet

You will know that I visited hypnotherapist Sue Bell soon after my homeopath Dr Bird. I saw an article about her and hypnotherapy and liked the sound of it. Perhaps it could help me overcome the doubts and fears of being so ill at such a young age. My first session with her was a new experience. She told me that it would be a form of relaxation and may help with my sleeping. It wouldn't cure my symptoms but help my mind deal with the ongoing situation. We did an experiment where she took me on a guided relaxation through all my body. Once in a deeply relaxed state, she began to gently tell my subconscious mind that I was feeling calm, confident and courageous. Many years later, I learned that the main beliefs and messages we live by are stored in our subconscious. She left me with a cassette recording that I was to play, every day, sitting in a chair for twenty minutes.

I came home and began to take this on board; it became a bit of a joke within our family. At first, I felt like it was being mocked, but after a while, I loved the whole thing and I didn't care. Every afternoon, I would clamber back upstairs to my bedroom if I had managed to get out of it and get dressed, which I certainly tried to do every day.

I used to say to Mum and Dad that I was going to do my hypnotherapy and didn't want to be disturbed. Thirty-six years ago, I was the first in my family to have been to hypnotherapy, so I was trailblazing here. I was creating a new way for myself but this also had an impact on those around me. I would sit in my grey chair, plug in my Walkman headphones, and click play on the cassette - yes, this was the 'old days' of cassettes! For twenty minutes, I would listen to hypnotherapist Sue, who asked me to deeply relax. As I continued with this practice, I found other relaxation and affirmation cassettes over the years. Having this time let my mind relax from all the worries and investigations; this was so crucial to my healing recovery.

I have continued to seek out different forms of relaxation over the years. With YouTube, the selection and accessibility now is vast.

This was the foundation stone of what I later termed 'P&Q'. The word 'meditation' is often used but I began to call this P&Q time. It has become a vital cocoon for me. I deeply feel that if we were all taught this from early on as children, we would be able to manage our nervous systems much better and self-soothe. We would gain clarity and wisdom from connecting to our higher selves and listening to the messages from within.

I learned more about the benefits of stillness and presence. Again, the nearest I had come to being aware of the concept of presence was immersed in piano practice or playing guitar.

After hypnotherapy, this was beginning to take on another meaning for me and I turned to researching what it was and how it may help me deal with the knock-on effects of my symptoms. I decided to visit an introductory meeting about Transcendental Meditation (TM) in the centre of Liverpool. The first problem to overcome was climbing up all the stairs to the meeting room at the top of a very old Georgian townhouse. After that meeting, I knew it would be really challenging to climb the stairs to the room; the price was also something to consider because I wasn't in a position to pay for the training. However, it sparked an interest in meditation, for this I am grateful.

Over the many years of meditating, I have discovered that TM is one type of meditation using a mantra given to you at the end of your one-to-one training. In this early stage, this wasn't where I turned; after hypnotherapy I began to use different tapes. One of the very first was Louise Hay's morning and evening practice, which I did for quite a long time, it was non-negotiable for me. I don't do it now, but if you are starting somewhere, it is a good place to start.

Call it meditation, call it quiet time, call it relaxation. It's code for stopping.

Creating a consistent 'quiet time', or 'stillness time' is a vital support system, to nurture and ground you. The word 'meditation' seems to conjure up all sorts of thoughts.

"I'm not that type of person."

"I don't have the time."

"I've tried it and it doesn't work."

"I can't sit cross legged."

"I'm no hippy."

Emptying your mind of all thoughts is actually a really difficult thing to do and so when it doesn't happen in the first few days, months, years, we believe we 'can't meditate', we give up and don't bother.

Meditation, stillness, and presence isn't about emptying the mind; the aim is to not attach to the thought that pops in. The purpose is to set aside quiet time every day to sit still and be still. Blocking off some time and space. What you do during the 'sitting still' can be up to you.

- Count breath cycles.
- Use one word and repeat the word e.g. c-a-l-m.
- Choose an affirmation.
- Introduce a Sanskrit mantra e.g. 'So Hum' (meaning 'I am').
- Listen to a chosen piece of music, only for this purpose, to anchor relaxation.
- Use apps such as Calm, or Headspace
- Melo; the small, guided device handheld breathing trainer

When thoughts fly in, hear yourself say 'thank you for that' and then bring yourself back to saying your word, phrase, mantra or begin the count again.

Carving out time in your day, every day, is taking responsibility, moving yourself further up your 'to-do list'. Choose to be still every morning before your day begins, or maybe find the space mid-morning, afternoon or early evening. You will find your way. Setting quiet time aside is an accumulative practice, doing it every day builds up within your body system and so if you miss one or two days, it won't be a terrible thing, but guess what, you'll discover ... you miss it.

It will be different for everyone, however, the gem of stillness and presence is finding the time and setting this aside as part of your daily practice.

Pause

The Magic Chair

In secondary school, we had a pastoral teacher, we called her Mrs C. She used to be the one you'd go to if you didn't feel well; she had a lovely, caring way about her. Her door was always open; you'd enter and tell her your woes, and she'd say, "*Come, come and sit in the magic chair.*" She'd give you half a paracetamol and encourage you on this very plain-looking random wooden 1960s chair where you would sit, quietly, watching her go about her day.

She may be having a conversational class in her room with pupils from another year. She'd just let you sit there quietly, she wouldn't push or ask you every two minutes how you felt. She'd leave you be.

In those ten minutes of peace and quiet, your symptoms would either be soothed, or not.

At the end, she would ask how you were and you'd either go back to class, or if feeling worse, you'd stay longer and she would arrange for a call to be made home. This always stuck with me. Mrs C and her magic chair. More often than not, those ten minutes of just peace and quiet, even in the midst of another babbly class, was just what I needed. It stuck with me.

So now I ask you ...

- Where is your magic chair?
- If you have no 'you' chair at home, is there a bench on the way to work, your local park, even your car.
- Do you want to seek out a self-hypnosis journey?
- Find a quiet spot and start with three minutes of P&Q.

I would avoid lying horizontal on the bed - you may fall asleep, the aim is not to fall asleep. Use music, if that helps, music that is new to you so you can set up a new pathway to the tune.

Start with three minutes and then build upon this, the most important thing here is to get into a rhythm, stop and find your magic chair and seek peace and quiet.

You may have a few magic chairs in different settings - the more the merrier.

Make P&Q a non-negotiable act every day and let your magic chair become an anchor to peace and quiet.

Co: No Means No

Saying no has always been something I have struggled with. I'm a yes girl. I love to help, I love to support and I don't want to disappoint. I have worked through many inner child issues, in therapy and on the page.

So, saying no didn't come easily or comfortably.

However, in the throes of ill health, I learned to say no because I had to look after myself.

No one else was going to look after me. Although my Mum was the first shield, I still took responsibility for me. I surrendered to taking baby steps forward; those steps were small and so tiny, I had to do something every day that gave me courage that I would get better.

Saying no was another baby step healing curve for me.

- I had to say no when people telephoned and I couldn't speak to them because I was so tired and had no energy to talk.

- I had to say no to invitations to weddings and engagement parties, because I had to conserve the little energy I had.
- I had to say no to food that wasn't going to help me feel stronger.
- I had to say no to people trying to help, who didn't really help, but were feeling guilty.
- I had to say no to tasks that drained me.
- I had to say no to holidays, trips out and car journeys that tired me and pushed my limits, taking five days to recover.
- I had to say no to family members and friends of family who thought I needed a push.
- I had to say no first, assess the situation and then reply.

I often backed myself into a very unrealistic corner if I said yes immediately.

- I had to learn to say yes to organise timings correctly based on what I knew my body could do, not what others thought I should be doing.
- I had to learn to say yes to the right kinds of people around me who wanted to support me, and be friends with me for the right reasons, rather than feeling sorry for me.
- I had to learn to say yes to going to the places and invitations that made my heart sing and no to all things that made me feel uncomfortable and pushed.

- I had to learn to say yes to spending time with family and friends of family who supported me and no to those that made me feel even more fatigued.
- I had to get used to saying no first, assessing and then responding.

No. Assess. Respond.

For someone who always said yes but without assessing, it was vital for my recovery.

Saying NO creates a cocoon around you, so that you realise that you are in control.

If you're struggling, balancing your health is a priority, putting yourself first, is not being selfish; it's time to create boundaries.

By the way, did you know you can also say NO after a YES?

Pause

Know your Compass

1. Do you say yes when really you mean no, and you get stuck in a corner?
2. Do you accept invitations that you know you can't accomplish?
3. Are you putting your own self on the back burner, thinking it will take care of itself (ps it won't).

What do you need to say no to and what's the best way of saying no that feels comfortable to you? How can you say it? Some examples I used to say.

- "Thanks so much, I will have to check on this one, can I call you back?"
- "No, I'm sorry, I won't be able to do that at the moment."
- "Please excuse me, I'm going to have to go now."
- "Thank you but no."

What other ways do you think you can say no, and more importantly, where do you need to start?

Co: Bedtime Ritual

One of the best pieces of advice I received from one of the consultants I saw was to make sure I was in bed, lights out by 10.00 p.m., definitely before 10.30 p.m.

Although I was always tired and coping with extreme fatigue and exhaustion, I didn't have the best sleep pattern. I often either couldn't get to sleep or I would sleep at the wrong time of the day from sheer tiredness and then when it came to sleeping at night, it wouldn't be easy at all and I would wake up a couple of times. I had to cope with my symptoms, which really impacted my sleep.

Now I start making my way to bed around 9.30 p.m., sometimes, it may be 9 p.m. I am not a big TV watcher so I'll be reading, talking, video calling, playing with my dogs, writing, getting into bed and flowing through a mantra to sleep after taking some homeopathic remedies that have been really helping me in recent times. There are several pieces of music that I play; particular mantras from Deva Premal, sounds of the ocean, solfeggio frequencies, gongs, Tibetan bowls, crystal bowls, all help to soothe.

My goal is for me to turn out the light by 10.30 p.m. and this piece of advice I have always kept in mind. Sometimes it happens, sometimes it doesn't. I make sure that I follow the ritual at least four nights. It also depends on season; I may be more flexible in the lighter months.

Something happens with the brain when you create a ritual around flowing to sleep and especially trying to get to bed before midnight. It can begin to conserve energy rather than having to pull on the reserves to get you through this stress of pushing. I also would not eat anything late at night so that my digestive system is not having to work through the night to process those items. There is so much more to this and I'm not the expert, but for the purpose of this Way, examine whether you need more support.

Young mums and those of you with extra commitments at night, I would say that if you can create just two of these nights before 11, your body will thank you for it. With nursing children, you are dictated by their sleep patterns so it's important to sleep when they sleep if you can, and you have the support around you to do that.

Pause

Flow to Sleep

How can you create some ritual around being in bed ready for lights out at 10.30 p.m.

If you're usually a 2 a.m. lights out individual, chances are this is going to be a radical change for you, however your body will thank you for it. Managing on five hours of sleep a night is not a good start to the day, our body would prefer more and if we are feeling run down, tired, out of sync, then it's important to begin this shutdown and create a sacred space around going to bed. Think about an eye mask to cut out sensory stimulation.

So what can *you* do?

Do you need to reach out for support?

Depending on your life situation, can you think of a few ways that would make you 'flow into sleep?'

What is your body, mind and spirit asking for?

Turn quietly to your journal and see if there are any whispers.

Co: Electronics and EMF

I didn't have mobile technology to deal with back in the 90s. However, I still took a break from watching television and listening to music or radio. The type of music I listened to and the quality of the movies and documentaries was very important. I always knew I needed to switch off from any radio wave technology. I suppose that was the intuitive me, calling me.

Over the last twenty years, we have seen technology become what is being referred to as The Fourth Industrial Revolution. Technology is in every facet of our lives and we have fallen under its spell, it serves us but we are also serving it. There is rapid expansion within industries and our day-to-day life and societal patterns. This includes and is not exclusive:

- Mobile communication masts all over the cities.
- 5G towers.
- Wi-Fi pounding through everybody's home.
- More wireless connections to boilers, electric

meters, heating systems, Alexa, Siri, Ring, alarm systems etc.

- Mobile phones include smartphones and pads with instant access to communications.

So this is a modern-day cocoon from my experience in the last ten years as things have unfolded.

Let's just start with Wi-Fi signals in our homes and all around us.

As vibrational beings with our own biofield, of magnetic and electric pulsation, our bodies are constantly bombarded with man made 'radio waves' all around us and it can be quite energy depleting, if we are already feeling low and run down.

As I am always fundamentally looking at removing stressors and pressures from my body, mind and spirit to enable restoration and self-healing, I began to explore reverting to using an ethernet cable at home for my desktop; however, it was always something I grappled with because I too have become dependent on wireless technology. Therefore, I began with turning off the router in my home so that my body has time to replenish during the night while sleeping. I was also very aware of where my router was located and if in my office studio, was I spending all day sitting right next to it.

Otherwise, I feel like I'm constantly 'on'. Radiating. Buzzing.

Here are some other things that I do that I find helps me.

- Having a twenty-four hour electronic free day - this means no phone, laptop, TV. Taking a break.
- Creating electronic free times e.g., using my laptop

during certain hours and not after a certain time or not taking it into my bedroom.

- Not having my laptop on my knee with the power cord connected.
- Keeping my smart phone out of my bedroom and not charging it there.
- Checking the radiation frequency emitted on my phone and wireless devices.
- Not having a TV in the bedroom.
- Switching off Wi-Fi routers and extension plug-ins at night.

This was all quite a challenge for me, I love my technology. I work in the online world a great deal, yet I find when I make a concerted effort to have this electronic fast, it feels freeing, releasing and balancing. You know the kind of feeling when you're on holiday and you have no signal and you're really bummed out but it takes you a couple of days to realise that it's a good thing.

Wherever all your technology is based, they will be emitting a frequency that is static and interfering, the same goes for how close you are to telecommunication masts near your home.

An incredible array of research shows links between health problems and electromagnetic frequencies. This topic is huge and one where we can personally investigate if our health is being impacted. It is often overlooked.

Fifteen years ago, I was at a four day workshop and one of the participants asked the facilitator if the router at the venue could be turned off during the day as she was greatly affected by the frequencies. It gave her very strong symptoms, for example, tiredness, headaches, lethargy and sore throats and she therefore wouldn't be able to stay for the day.

We need to counteract these high beaming frequencies with grounding and earthing, so this is a valuable tool here.

Pause

Tech Fast

Do you sense your WiFi being on all the time is draining you? At home and at work, have a look around, what is surrounding you; e.g., Smart TV's, Smart Meters, Ring doorbells, Alexa, laptops, smartphones, iPads, to name a few, what else is there? Wireless boilers, intruder alarms?

- Where is your router located?
- Can you test to see how much radiation is emitted?
- Maybe consider turning of your router at night while you sleep.
- Do you feel you can go with an electronic fast?
- Find options to counter balance the radiation emitted: e.g. protection

Start here.

The fifth Way

Create

to bring (something) into existence;
cause (something) to happen as a result of one's actions.

When I looked back through my old journals, I saw reconnecting with my creative self helped me so much. I knew that Create had to become a Way. In the creative art and craft space I was able to shift the focus of what I was dealing with daily. Intuitively, I began to visualise myself looking well, being healthy and full of vitality even though the present-day self wasn't, I tried somehow to feel how the future Julia would be; that's where I began to learn about visioning. Colour was a way to calm my mind and this played out in many ways, colouring-in being one of them, it connected me back to my childhood, and I later discovered the benefits of colouring in for adults. I instinctively began to build a deck of soothing cards that would lift up my day and find routes to creatively elevate my vibe through film joy. I would use the Way of Create to discover inspirational things to get me through my ill health and it powered me on, giving me something to hang on to when all else was feeling grim. Being creative is not about being artistic. We are all creators, it is in everything we are, in everything we do and everything we feel, it is our birthright and is available to us all if we can step out of our pre-conditioning.

Cr: Shift the Focus

My first niece was born when I was twenty-one years old. I was *The Happiest AJ Ever* (Aunty Julia). I couldn't wait to meet her. Here I was at the beginning of an awful time with my health problem and along came Niecey Number One, she massively shifted the focus.

It gave me an idea. Mum had some blank tapestry canvas left over, so I decided to have a go and draw a design of Winnie the Pooh and Piglet against a tree, using up the wool she had to make a framed tapestry for the nursery. This took me a while to do as I only had the energy to do a little bit at a time, some days more and other days, none. But I was pleased to be 'doing something.' It reconnected me to some part of myself that I had forgotten about – being creative.

> I can let go here with this tapestry - will it weave away the pain?

It had been nearly one year since I came home ill with flu, I was feeling so low. It felt unfair, unjust and I was still trying to find out what was wrong with me. In the meantime, I became engrossed in this creative tapestry activity where I could, while watching Around The World in 80 Days with Michael Palin.

> Through his travels I feel like I am going somewhere! C'mon Jules, Shift The Focus.

I needed to immerse myself into something that was not connected to my situation - my health dictated what I could and couldn't do, because of time and stamina. However, I felt so strongly, even back then, that if I was able to shift the focus from my ill health even for a short while to something else, maybe learning something new, reading a different book, or trying a new craft, by giving myself a creative leg-up, my body, mind and soul felt uplifted.

Not long after this epic first tapestry, I received a book voucher as a gift and on a trip to my local bookstore with Mum, I was instantly (and I mean instantly) drawn to a book called The Complete Book of Beads by Janet Coles. I was mesmerised.

There and then, I fell in love with the colours of the beads, their country of origin, the tools you need to make necklaces, earrings, and bracelets. It was another creative outpouring, channelling into the Fifth Way of Create.

I did a little at a time, based on my energy levels, but as my health progressed in the right direction over the years, this creative outpouring became something that fulfilled me and I was able to contemplate having tables at coffee mornings and little craft fairs. I couldn't do them on my own, but it provided me with a creative outlet.

Dog Grooming

Benjie, our adorable family dog, who had been with us for about two years, was always near me and although I couldn't walk him in the very early years, he became my best mate and helped me shift the focus. He was a long-haired dog, so when I had more energy at my disposal, I would brush him; if I had a 'good' hour, I would clip him with our clippers. I had to teach myself how to do it, I loved doing it. It took some skill and on one of the first attempts I forgot to put the clipper attachment on and gave him a Mohican stripe right up the middle of his beautiful fur... so I had to cut more than I would have liked so he didn't look so strange! I didn't do that again.

Art

I have always been artistic and loved art and design throughout my childhood and even in secondary school, I studied O-Level Art from fourteen to sixteen years old. I would get treated to supplies for birthdays and holiday presents. One in particular was a set of pastels - a whole new medium for me. I loved creating landscapes and was captivated by drawing birds. An elderly couple who lived opposite us, brought over a couple of beautifully illustrated bird books and left them with me. How did she know? Was that Mum weaving her magic by asking her? She knew I was very poorly from Mum. I had no formal training with pastels but I just enjoyed the medium and the mess, I let it flow. I didn't worry about getting things right or in proportion I loved colour and creating my own version of these birds.

As Julia Cameron, author of The Artist's Way wrote *"Art is therapeutic, not therapy."*

Sewing

Niecey Number Two and Niecey Number Three came along quite swiftly. I was AJ again and again within two yearly intervals, which happened in these early years of ill health; what a beautiful way to shift the focus. On top of the original Winnie-the-Pooh tapestry, I made mobiles for cots, nappy stackers for nappies, stuffed dinosaurs, rag dolls, little taffeta dresses, t-shirts, sweatshirts, jewellery, decoupage door plaques. Those nieces of mine were a gift from the heavens as they helped me to shift the focus and explore my creative side.

All of the time when I was feeling so ill, I was thinking of what I could do when I had ten minutes where I felt okay. There were countless days when all I could do was lie in bed or on the couch, but in my mind, I thought of the next thing to 'shift the focus'.

I taught myself new skills and combined with all the other Ways, it felt like it was helping me such a great deal. Because of my health situation, when I accomplished a creative piece, whether it was a pair of earrings or a tapestry, it calmed my mind, soothed my soul and gave me confidence.

Pause

Follow the Cues

I'd like to encourage you to follow the creative cues and nudges - choose something that will shift the focus and if you're feeling okay, give yourself ten minutes a day to do something very different or learn something new, building this up to maybe thirty minutes.

Depending on how out of balance you feel, you will know the time you can allocate to this. Here are some ideas to consider:

- Take a photo a day of something or someone that makes you smile. Often when we focus on a collection of the same thing we build up a gallery of gratitude.
- Start a blog. It's easy to start writing your thoughts even for ten minutes. It can be on anything you choose.
- Learn to knit or crochet.
- Learn a language and then listen and take part in a conversation.
- Complete a doodle-a-day with only a black marker pen and notebook.

... and when energy levels are a little higher.

Visit an arts and crafts store, take a trip down the children's aisle

- Make your first felt doll.
- Glass paint a wind chime.
- Decorate your own mug.
- Mosaic a place mat.
- Make your first ever candle.
- Decoupage over some paper mâché letters.
- Buy some blank cards and envelopes and create some cards to send out to your friends and family around the world using paper punches, pretty paper and stamps.
- Visit your local library and be pulled in by colourful books.

Shifting the focus boosts your inner levels of energy and helps your body, mind and spirit restore, it also helps you to let go and let flow and not think about your situation all the time. What other ideas are you having here?

Cr: Vision On

My life was on hold. I didn't know how long this was going to continue, my self-esteem was down the pan and my confidence ... well, let's put it this way, I had none. Being ill was robbing me of everything. I was desperate, I had limited reserves. Having a shower or washing my hair took every ounce of me. I was itching to look forward to a life that oozed wellness, I longed for a career that made me jump for joy and a relationship that shook my world, fulfilling and loving. I ached for travel and yearned for my own space again, because I was living back with my parents having had a two-year independence-break, working in the world of commerce in a different city. There were dreams, but I just couldn't see them properly. I was tired all the time, the dreams, well, they were fuzzy and deep, deep inside.

I had always been a rock steady journaller, head stuck in a notebook where possible and pen in hand, I had written tonnes of pages on finding my way through these health troubles and scratched out some desires and goals but I was completely stuck.

I couldn't see a way through.

I wanted to feel less anxious about the way my life was going. Looking around me, I saw other sufferers ill for 20 + years and I cried myself to sleep, hoping this was not going to be me. I was stressed out about the recovery statistics, I was flapping about which way to turn and my gut instinct and intuition were taking a real beating.

This idea kept growing inside of me that as well as writing in my journal, I would find a new blank notebook and rip out images and words from the magazines that I had piling up in my room. Images that inspired and motivated me. This became my little go-to task of the day, nothing fancy just ripping images with glue stick in hand. I didn't make big collages back then, it was just small and simple. I would rip and paste an image that my insides loved, a colour, a phrase, a word. If my gut instinct loved it, I'd rip it out.

I recognised after a few months that this little practice was boosting my inner spirit, it gave me a lift.

I began to see similar images popping out, animals featured a lot, dogs in particular, craft, art, making, design, bright colours, scenes from nature, travel, words that were big and bold, things like 'do it, lush, loving, boss' I felt a sense of warmth growing deep in my belly, not sure what it was but it felt like – a knowing, somewhere amongst the pages, I could play in here, it was safe, fun and non-judgmental.

This very early visual notebook turned into a cool tool that let me hear whispers of my intuition, it showed me that I could give myself some space to dream. It soothed me when I felt exhausted drained and lifeless. I felt small nudges of what's next. I got to see a visual cue of my soul and what I was desiring.

Fast forward to the present day and this has become a crucial part of my ReBalancing Toolkit that helps to recharge me and also my clients.

Now when I turn to magazines, glue stick and vision book, I truly recognise that this is a beautiful mindfulness practice. I find my breathing slows down, I begin to feel differently about where I'm at and where I want to be. I feel braver. I feel calmer. I feel less stressed about what's happening around me and I can feel the rumblings of transformation.

As I create these empowering spirit loving vision books, I can see the map of my inner world emerging.

I can choose to follow these maps and be guided by the imagery and words, or I can just experience the beautiful process I have just had, allowing the imagery and words to connect to my intuitive know-how.

I focused on how I wanted to feel in my life after I got well, deep down I had to believe that I was going to get well, and I wanted to 'picture' a Julia in the future who was well, happy, fulfilled and content, doing what she loved and living in a healthy way with possibly a husband and kids. This was something I focused upon even when times were extremely tough.

Mum asked our local hairdressers for their magazines; family, friends would bring any over and I would flip through them and rip out images and words that made me feel:

- Joyful. Contented. Fulfilled.
- Calm. Relaxed. Creative. Crafty.
- Enthusiastic. Energised. Full of Vitality.

Doing this was difficult when I didn't 'feel' these feelings, but I wanted to, so I stepped into the visual image.

When I cut or ripped out images and words, I allowed myself time to contemplate and visualise how I saw my future self.

Creating these visuals was not about being creative and it wasn't about being artistic. Being relaxed and feeling my future self was where I wanted to begin. During my healing journey, I built upon these smaller inspirational books to develop larger vision books and even vision walls, this has grown over the decades and you will often find me creating a vision page.

Pause

Imagining You

This is a map of your world and more so a map of what you're imagining. You can make it any size you want.

Gather stacks of magazines. Don't think too much about type/style, go with what is attracting you. Find a hairdresser who will give you a pile or ask at the library. If you can, include a picture of yourself somewhere in the vision book, board/wall.

Spend some time cutting or ripping out images that appeal to you. You can do this whichever way you want: some people spend a little time cutting/ripping, gathering a selection, then paste with glue when they have a good stash. I like doing it this way, but if I'm reading a magazine and see something, I'll rip it out and stick it there and then. Go with your intuition when you see certain images and words, avoid analysing or thinking too deeply about what you're picking, or whether it's 'right.'

Collect your supplies:

- Glue stick.
- Scissors.
- Washi Tape (for your book/board and wall).
- Plain notebook either large A3 or A4, or if you want to do one board, choose size A2 or even A1.
- Blue Tack (if creating a vision wall).

I want you to go to your visions to lose yourself in those images and you can think, see, feel, hear what it would be like to “be in it”. This could become a daily practice, cutting and sticking images that resonate with the way you want your future you to FEEL.

You can choose to do a generic vision page, or decide to focus on a particular area for example:

Wealth, abundance and prosperity
Career, job, and working life.
Love, intimacy and relationships.
Friendships, fun, laughter, and interests.
Health and wellness.
Creativity, joy, and inner contentment.
Travel and independence.
Knowledge, learning, and development.
Spirituality, peace, and tranquillity.

Or you may want to include ALL of these in your vision pages and board.

What messages are coming forward for you through the imagery and words?

Cr: Colour Spectrum

Someone gifted me a colouring book when I was ill. It took me straight back to childhood when I was very ill with tonsillitis; all I wanted to do was colour in. Mum would always say that she would know when I was starting with a sore throat as I would intuitively get out my colouring book and felt-tip pens; she knew that something was brewing. So here I was stepping back into the space where colour began to soothe me.

> I find it so very therapeutic.

This is an important Way that I have always used from the little Julia to the grown-up Julia, aged twentyish, who was trying to find out what was going on and restoring her health. The colour spectrum helped to create space within me, and light on the page, nurturing something that had a positive outcome. Even if it was for ten minutes.

Turning to colouring became a way to channel ill health -

whether I had a virus in bed, tonsillitis, coping with a cold, chicken pox or flu - there would never be a time when my colouring book and my pencil case full of Berol felt pens would not be far away from me. I also used to love the A1 posters you got called DoodleArt, which came with a pack of ten Berol pens - it used to take me ages to complete but I would love them.

Colouring enabled me to 'zone out' and immerse myself in something else that wasn't about being ill.

The colours soothed me. The scenes mesmerised me. The motion of colouring transported me to other times.

I doodled; I created shapes.

Words, flowers, trees, hearts, angels, teddy bears, dogs.

I found books to colour in or I spent time doodling in a plain white sketchbook, colouring as I went along.

This was not about being an artist; this was picking up pens and colour and allowing myself to be taken into a colouring meditation of stillness and presence.

On a deeper level this is inner child heart work.

I know from working with clients in private practice and having been in therapy myself, connecting to our inner child helps to heal and look after the small child within us. Our inner child has many parts and colouring in tapped into my free-spirited creative, little Julia.

Just the other day, I was in the art store and I overheard an elderly lady asking if there were any colouring in books for adults as her husband was at home poorly and he asked her to buy him some felts and a colouring book. I knew that this confirmed that I was not wrong about the power of colouring. I turned to her to join in the admiration for colouring and she told me he always turned to it when he was having an unwell day.

When I delved more into the colour spectrum, I discovered that it contains a range of colours according to their electromagnetic wavelength, from the shortest to the longest. Therefore, colour is light vibrating at certain speeds. The visible colour spectrum that we humans see is the rainbow; red, orange, yellow, green, blue, indigo, violet. Lower light vibrations produce warmer colours like the reds and oranges, higher vibrations produce cooler colours like blues and indigo. At the highest vibration, the two ends of the colour spectrum meet together and produce violet. It is no coincidence that these seven colours also match the chakra system; each colour resonates and supports different areas of our bodies.

According to Collins Dictionary, the spectrum is the range of different colours produced when light passes through a glass prism or a drop of water. A rainbow shows the colours in the spectrum, to the human eye.

Chakras are associated with energy, so each one carries a unique frequency and wavelength. The colour assigned to every chakra is specifically chosen to match the vibration of that particular energy centre.

'Each of these [chakras] in the temple of the body is designed to handle a particular kind of energy. Moreover, each chakra greatly affects the mind, body, and spirit in its own unique way, just as colours do. To really comprehend the chakra colours and their meaning, it helps to understand colour in general.' Anodea Judith, trainer of Mindvalley's Chakra Healing Quest.

Therefore, choosing colours when colouring takes on a whole new meaning.

Pause

Colouring in

There has been a big resurgence of adult colouring, so you can find several books to colour. If you're wishing to tap into your inner child, perhaps an A1 style of poster could be the right thing. Find felts that you love and just begin. Mandalas can be incredibly soothing, whether drawing them from scratch or a colouring in book.

Perhaps you want to create doodles to colour - buy yourself an A5 sketchbook that has crisp white paper, a black sharpie and some felts and start to create shapes, curves, waves, swirls and begin to colour. See what you can see in the shapes. Patterns begin to emerge and you'll be mesmerised and transported into another meditative state.

I published Muse Mantra Colouring Meditations in 2018; this is a lovely journal-style meditative book which was the culmination of working in a group of women, drawing seventy-six of them and their mantra. Muse Mantras can be used as powerful totems and talismans in your day-to-day life, in healing spaces, on altars, in stillness and presence rooms, they are also being used as prompts to write in journals, placed on vision boards, stuck in visual books and even as bookmarks. Why not use the colouring experience to create a calm moment in your daily life, it is proven that colouring can help alleviate tension and stress in adults.

Cr: Soothing Deck

My first initiation into making a soothing card deck was at this time. I turned to finding phrases, prayers, song lyrics, quotes, all to inspire, soothe and calm me. Although I tried to stay positive about everything, there were days of doubt as I felt such a lack of confidence about my health. I wanted to turn my mind from what was happening in my day-to-day situation and turn inwards. These cards helped me with 'a card for the day,' giving me something to journal about, talk about if it sparked another idea, or contemplate if things challenged me.

I turned to making them when I felt I could. I kept all the supplies in a dedicated box, so I just needed to pick up this box and get creative. In the end with my little stash, I found a cute little fabric bag to keep them in and they were never too far away from me. It inspired me to look at other inspirational card decks, buying a few in the years following. I used card decks as prompts for inner reflection, contemplation and journalling and found I would also use them in my P&Q practice to focus on one word within a prayer, or a specific lyric, or mantra. I went on to create my own card deck, The Muse Mantra Deck, a deck of fifty cards with affirmations on them, sold around the world, these are used in therapy rooms, yoga classes and for individuals who want to feel inspired.

Pause

Cards Lift Up

Here is how I created mine; why not think about creating a set for yourself?

I bought a sheet of A1 white card stock and cut this up to be the size of a business card (approximately 3.5 inches x 2 inches/8.9 x 5.1 cm).

You can also now buy small packs of white cards that are already pre-cut. I made forty of them.

- On ten, I wrote prayers that I sought from different biblical, mystical, philosophical texts and inspiring books.
- On ten, I wrote lines from song lyrics that really resonated with me.
- On ten, I wrote quotes that inspired and soothed me.
- On one, I wrote YES
- On one, I wrote NO
- On one, I wrote I Love You Julia
- On one, I wrote What do you hear?

For that initial deck I decorated the back of each card differently, which I later discovered was not the best way of keeping the cards consistent. Later on I realised that the backs needed to look the same, but I loved them anyway.

Before or after my daily P&Q time, I would shuffle these little cards and choose one to see what appeared for me on that day. What I found was that I would intuitively pull a card that had something to do with what was going on for me at that time. The process of creating them was lovely; we don't need to be artistic to achieve this, it can be something that comes from within us and is an expression of our inner child. Remember the time when you used to love playing with crafty kits?

Jot down here any quotes, prayers, and lyrics that pop into your mind as you read this, to remind you for later.

Cr: Shift the Focus

What elevated my vibe were films that made me laugh, these became a form of therapy for me. I would seek them out via our local video shop (yep, I know!) when I was feeling a little stronger for a trip there. Friends would lend me videos they had and my mum would also bring some back from the library when I was very poorly.

I was open to films about positivity, fun, laughter, romance and smiles. In those days, we didn't have YouTube; now, it's a different story and when you're not on your tech fast, laughing and feeling joyful through films can really support your rebalancing process. It may seem incredibly obvious but exploring new films can be a tonic.

Below is a list of joy films to elevate your vibe, you may very well have more to add, it's lovely to keep a playlist for this very purpose. The films below have storylines with messages, some make us laugh and some make us cry; keep ones that resonate nearby and turn to them when you need to elevate your vibe.

The same can be said for music and comedy, so replicate this for music and comedy clips.

Amelie
Life of Pi
Chocolat
Win Win
The Shift
Vanilla Sky
Miss Potter
Mamma Mia
Funny Face
The Secret
Last Holiday
Dirty Dancing
Eat Pray Love
Field of Dreams
Roman Holiday
Stealing Beauty
Wings of Desire
Hideous Kinky
The Tree of Life
Love Actually
Saving Grace
Pay it forward
Little Children
What About Me
Carry on Films
A Good Year
The Proposal
The Holiday

Safe Haven
The Goonies
Life in a Day
Say Anything
The Notebook
A Knight's Tale
The Fisher King
The Lucky One
Valentine's Day
As It Is In Heaven
Definitely, Maybe
Laurel and Hardy
Good Will Hunting
Where the Heart Is
Monsoon Wedding
It's a Wonderful Life
Fisherman's Friends
Truly, Madly, Deeply
The Joy Luck Club
Cyrano de Bergerac
A Room with a View
Dances with Wolves
Under the Tuscan Sun
The Cider House Rules
The Darjeeling Limited
You Can Heal Your Life
Like Water for Chocolate
What Dreams May Come
The Pursuit of Happyness
I Am Love (with Tilda Swinton)
Coco Chanel & Igor Stravinsky

The Tape with Martha Tilston
No Arms, No Legs, No Worries
What the Bleep Do We Know!?
The Best Exotic Marigold Hotel
Cheerful Weather for the Wedding
2 Days in Paris/2 Days in New York
Sweet November (with Keanu Reeves)
Eternal Sunshine of the Spotless Mind
Bright Star (directed by Jane Campion)

Pause

Film Joy

What films can you add to the above?

Perhaps also create a list of Music Joy and Comedy Joy.

You may also want to note the feelings you felt when watching some of the films above.

Use phrases and songs within the films as prompts in your journal, to dig deeper and self reflect.

The Sixth Way

Move

a change of place, position, or state,
an act that initiates or advances a process or plan.

During the acute years of my ill health, being able to move was incredibly difficult. My energy stores were depleted, embarking on movement was significantly limited. I had to review what 'move' meant. In those early years it became an internal move and when my stamina flickered, I was able to initiate an external move. Back in the days of my health restoration, I would ask myself, could I move in another way? If I was feeling heavy and very stuck because of low energy, I would create a new affirmation which I wrote out multiple times. This made me move – internally. If I was feeling overwhelmed with all my symptoms, I would turn to box breathing, helping me to stay present in my day, calming my mind, soothing my soul. When I was able to move externally, I would turn to tai chi, beginning with a slow-moving exercise to feel energy present in my hands or qi gong where I would shake my hands and body. Finally, if I needed to let go of something bothering me at any point, I would turn to letter writing. The tools in this Way are for internal and external moving. As my health began to restore and balance, I would turn to Pilates, yoga and walking, in addition to rebounding and belly dancing.

This Way is an option for you to consider - contemplate

how you move. Move has always been a big area that I struggled with during these years, because it was to do with energy levels and post exercise malaise; I later discovered that this was to do with the being extremely hyper-mobile. I had to reframe what moving meant. In all the years of ill health, my leg muscles became less strong - now in my fifties I am still working on strengthening, the left-over ramifications of being ill for so long has taken its toll. I am still trying to crack the code.

M: Affirm

Did you ever have to write lines when you were in school? It used to fall upon you if you were naughty or doing something the teacher thought was 'bad.' The punishment would be to write ten, twenty, sometimes fifty lines.

My teacher used to tell me to write this one a lot:

I must not talk in class.

When I was in the throes of feeling so unwell, I would turn to 'lines' helping me to move through the pain both internally and externally, it helped me to balance whatever was going on in my mind and body. Only this time was different, I flipped them and used them in a good way.

A year or so later, I learnt that these were called 'affirmations' and within her book You Can Heal Your Life, Louise Hay shares much more about them and how to write them and later on Barefoot Doctor, Stephen Russell, wrote a book about affirmations, Manifesto: How To Get What You Want Without Trying where he explores more about the art of writing affirmations.

Affirmations are ways to open the door to our subconscious mind; every thought we think speaks to our inner selves, and if that is affirming a repeated negative message, we are creating a negative stream. We are confirming what we believe about ourselves and our lives, in repetition. I began to pay attention to what I was telling myself and the spelling I was using. Words have power. It's called spell - ing for a reason.

I was learning that I was (and am) a conscious creator and by rephrasing the messages to myself that I was playing over and over, I could assist the reprogramming of my subconscious mind.

I never berated myself, I was following what I was seeing throughout my life, school, community, family and friends. People throughout the years have said affirmations don't work, which means that maybe they haven't been explained effectively. As Louise Hay wrote, '*Affirmations are like seeds planted in soil. Poor soil, poor growth. Rich soil, abundant growth. The more you choose to think thoughts that make you feel good, the quicker the affirmations work.*'

So I began to write:

Every area of my health is in balance.
I am calm, confident and full of vitality now.
I am my best friend and I care for myself daily.

I used to write these in multiple-line format, I would also do these on post-it notes and place them around my mirror or in a place that I would see regularly. By writing lines I was sending the message directly to my subconscious mind by repeating them over and over again. Ultimately I would flip into a new statement if and when I heard myself say something that was contrary to what I was feeling. This has been and always will be an ongoing practice for me.

“Can I start thinking about my future?

Pause

Flip The Lines

What you have been saying to yourself over and over? Note down any statements that come to the forefront of your mind and you hear yourself say on a regular basis. Examples may be:

> My body feels sore and painful.
>
> I am overweight, it makes me feel so sad.
>
> My house is dark and stifling.
>
> This is so overwhelming; I don't know which way to turn.
>
> Now let's flip them:
>
> My body feels light and full of energy.
>
> I feel fit, healthy and full of vitality, I feel joy all around me.
>
> Every day in every way, I feel peace and light in my home.
>
> I seek out the possibilities and use my intuition.

Choose how many times you want to write your lines every day: ten, twenty, thirty. Record the flipped lines into an audio app, play them back, first thing on waking and last thing at night as you drift off to sleep. These times of the day are where the veil between waking and sleeping is thin.

M: Calm Your Nerves

It didn't take me long to realise that breathing was vital to healing. This wasn't about my practise of stillness and presence at that time (although that has changed over the past thirty years), but the breath itself was crucial. Breathing from the chest and not from the belly can often be a chronic fatigue and tiredness symptom. Was I hyperventilating? I began to notice if I was breathing through my mouth and from my upper chest in very quick successive breaths.

One of the things I had noticed in dealing with the constant fatigue was the incapacity to get back to 'normal life', which made me feel anxious. Everything was happening so slowly. The question of 'what is normal' is a big question which I won't attempt to answer now.

It seemed like it was taking such a long time to get well. Yet I had to keep going. When reading about it, I knew that I had to calm my nervous system; it was my mind that could gently support my physical body and, subsequently my spirit, helping me to restore my vitality.

I turned to a breathing technique called box breathing. Here, I would breathe in for a count of four, hold for four, exhale for four and hold for four. All done through the nose. I completed this cycle four times or however many I felt drawn to complete. I soon realised how powerful it was for me to be still and focus on my breath. Later I also learned that breathing out for a count slightly longer than breathing in calmed the parasympathetic nervous system. For example, breathing in for a count of four and breathing out for six.

This became one way to quieten my monkey chatter mind.

I either lay in bed, or if I could, I sat in my grey chair where I felt nurtured and supported and let myself explore my breath. The aim here is to cultivate this skill so that you can do it anywhere and at any time.

Pause

Box Breathing

How do you breathe? Do you take short sharp intakes of breath or breathe through your mouth while asleep?

Let's begin to learn Box Breathing through your nose only. Can you find yourself a quiet space, a magic chair, somewhere you will not be disturbed? Your car? The bathroom? Under a tree?

- Inhale for the count of four
- Hold for four.
- Exhale for four.
- Hold for four.
- Inhale for four.
- Repeat four times.

As you breathe in, expand your belly, see how far you can push it out. You will be cajoling your diaphragm into breathing deeply, something it may not have done for a while. Being mindful about breathing is one of the ways to move back to centre and balance.

M: Feel the Sphere

There were many days that I just couldn't physically move. I didn't have the energy.

I could barely have a shower some days and washing my hair was the day's task on some of those bad days. I loved swimming but getting there was an epic feat: undress, get in the pool, swim-ish, get out of the pool, shower, get dressed, then home. I knew that movement was important for me but I was wondering where I could find a smoother kind of movement and what it would look like.

It was then I came across tai chi. It was a very small class local to me, I phoned the teacher and explained my health problems, he said it would be fine for me to sit in a chair and just do what I could. Whether that would be to lift my arm or turn my head. However, when I went, I didn't have the stamina to cope with the session because, of course, I had to get there, climb the few stairs and be surrounded by people; my energy level didn't have the extra oomph for this. It really was dire in those very early days.

Yet I kept positive that I would find my way through this maze.

I explained to the teacher that I just couldn't see myself going at that time every week, so I asked if there were any exercises I could do at home. He introduced me to an exercise that was very gentle, that I could do sitting or lying down - it would start to move the energy around my body. I can't recall the name of it but I called it, 'The Ball of Chi' because one of my oldest childhood friends is called Chi. I felt soothed by the ball of chi. I always turn to this exercise whenever I need calm, whether I have been working at my desk for too long or boiling the kettle and need to feel soothed.

Fast forward fifteen years later, when I was fully well, I was excited to finally learn the entire Yang Short Form by attending Barefoot Doctor's Tai Chi retreat in Wales. It was the most exhilarating experience to be taught the form on a hillside in a very mixed climate. I feel so immensely proud of myself that I was able to stand there and learn the entire short form. Barefoot Doctor, Stephen Russell was a close friend of mine and whom I travelled to various tai chi weekends and retreats, along with organising events for him, sadly, he passed away suddenly in January 2020, his wisdom is always around me.

Pause

The Ball of Chi

With your hands outstretched, imagine you are resting your palms on a ball about the size of a small football; imagine a real-life ball there.

- Close your eyes and begin to move your hands around it to keep it moving.
- Once you start to do this, you will feel the tingle between both palms.

This is your biofield/energy field, the electricity that you produce from your electrical and magnetic body. This is soothing, warming, healing; you can move this around your body, up your arms, over your head, and feel the connectivity between the biofield of your energetic body and the energy around you.

In those early days, I would start off and do this for thirty seconds and gradually build it up.

This can become extremely meditative and is a very moving practise.

M: Shake it Out

While studying for my degree in health, I was moving positively up and out of my illness. During this time I took an elective module about complementary health approaches and I decided to seek out a community clinic I had heard of in Liverpool offering auricular acupuncture. This clinic was set up with funding to help the community with stress management, post-traumatic stress, pain management, mental and emotional balance, detoxification, addiction, substance misuse, and general well-being. It became very attractive asset where individuals would pop into the clinic for a 'pinning', where a NADA Practitioner inserted up to five needles in each ear for up to twenty five minutes while clients sat in a relaxed atmosphere, drinking detox tea and enjoying the company of all other ages in their community.

I loved this whole concept and I went on to train in the NADA protocol. NADA stands for National Acupuncture Detoxification Association. Initially, this was established in 1985 for help with substance misuse and detoxification by Dr

Michael Smith, Director of the Lincoln Recovery Centre, New York, and in 1988 John Tindall introduced it to the UK and established the Yuan Traditional Medicine College. It was with John that I did my training.

Why the ear?

Like reflexology for the hands and feet, the ear also has a complete map of the body system. Using auricular acupuncture, the outer ear acts like a switchboard that sends impulses to the brain, stimulating the release of endorphins that lower stress and induce relaxation.

On our first training day, John introduced us to a qi gong exercise and had us all standing up shaking out the chi (energy). I recognised that intuitively I did something along those lines in my first few years; it can be done very gently depending on your energy levels. It is a great exercise to do to step away from the computer screen and one I have integrated into my life over the years.

Pause

Get Chiqi

This is a very straightforward exercise to do, it can be very helpful when processing bad news, an anxious experience, or to just feel a change. It actually reminds me of my two dogs who shake at various times; when they wake after a sleep, when they're playing to share how they're feeling with each other, when they're moving through a stressful time or after a shock. Most creatures shake.

- Stand with your feet shoulder-width apart, feet flat on the floor.
- Ensure your knees are bent slightly, not locked, but some flexibility there; back is straight, bottom tucked in and forward.
- Stand with your arms relaxing at your sides.
- Begin by raising on to the balls of your feet and then down on your heels. As you land, begin shaking your body gently, from the wrists, to neck, to knees, be gentle, especially with your neck, no quick moves here.
- Breathe in and out from your diaphragm, expelling air through your teeth, or nose if you prefer. Shake slowly.
- Relax and bounce. Practise this for a full minute.

M: Letter it Go

In the early days at home, I wrote letters. Lots of letters! These were the days before email; it was a way for me to reach out and connect to friends and family around the world. There was nothing quite like receiving a letter through the post. However, I remember learning about writing a letter to my younger self through a counsellor. I know now that this was a very healing way to care for myself and release whatever was in my heart and mind. So, when I had the oomph I would write letters to little Julia, teenage Julia and older, wiser, healed Julia.

I wrote letters to people from my past who had died, upset me or I deeply loved and those from my present.

I never sent any of the letters but burnt them outside in a terracotta pot - I thought I was a little strange doing it but it was intuitive to do - I didn't want anyone to find the letters. Now I know that this is a ritual from ancient ceremonies.

Releasing the words: forgiving, forgiveness, sadness, anger.

Inviting in new words: love, vitality, health, wellness, harmony, peace, calm, joy.

All I ever needed was a pen and a pad. This was a way to move emotions through me, to nurture whatever was being held, to release and move forward. The internal move here can be quite significant.

An emotion is Energy-in-Motion.

Let go and let flow.

> “Feeling like I’m going to beat this and come out of the tunnel, wiser, happy, healthy and enjoying life - went to a party for the first time in 4 years.

Pause

Dear Dot Dot Dot...

When you read Letter it Go, who pops into your mind? Do you want to write to yourself? If so, what age? Do you wish to write a letter to a friend or family member to tell them how you're feeling or what you're seeking? Is there someone who has died or someone who has hurt you?

Grab yourself something to write with and paper you won't mind burning or ripping up, and start.

Dear ...

When you have written from your heart, find an envelope, you can write their name on it or a symbol, wait till you feel the time is right to burn it. Sometimes it's good to re-read your words, other times, not, you will know. There is no right or wrong. Set up some time alone, allocate a clay pot. As you begin to light one corner of your envelope, say to yourself:

I release all the words within this letter. I let my words dissipate and dissolve and transform any negative feelings and emotions back to nature, into the earth. Grant me courage to move forward, with vitality, with love, with joy, with peace. So be it.

Extra Ways

Over the past twenty-five years since rebalancing my health and healing from ME, I went further into the field of health and wellbeing. I immersed myself into many approaches both personally and professionally, teaching in further and higher education, therapeutic spaces, training within business settings, and establishing my holistic health private practice. Throughout those years, I have been inspired to continue my learning and development, critically assessing and integrating more and more into my daily life.

I delved more into consciousness, quantum physics, epigenetics, metaphysics, frequency, vibration and sound. Here, I felt like I had found a key to a secret that had stayed hidden.

At the time of writing The Way of the Boomerang, I began to reflect upon whether I would include these extra ways; they weren't what I did in the early days, the thirty way points that assisted me with restoring and balancing were fundamentally what gently shifted my journey.

However, these that follow have become such very important additions for me over the decades, including them here gives you an opportunity to investigate further, experiment and experience yourself. So, let's map out what has continued to help me over the last twenty five years.

Sound Healing - Solfeggios/Hertz Frequencies

I had always been very interested in the power of sound for restoring health from early in my healing journey, recognising that music was soothing and mesmerising. It was an intuitive call. It wasn't until my late thirties that I began to look into the therapeutics of music, particularly the frequency connection and how this had been used over millennia to stimulate our self-healing capacity. I went to sound baths where I would lie warm and cosy with blankets and pillows, feeling the stimulus and resonance of huge gongs, crystal bowls, drums, koshi chimes, tuning forks, and Tibetan singing bowls to name just a few. I devoured this and went on to study the foundation in integrated sound therapies, which I could use in my private therapy practice, and I have quite a collection of instruments that I have built up over the years.

The Solfeggio Frequencies are a series of six electromagnetic musical tones that the Gregorian monks were said to use when they chanted in meditation. Rediscovered in 1974 by Dr Joseph Puleo, the Solfeggio Frequencies are said to deeply penetrate the conscious and subconscious mind, stimulating inner healing. Dr Puleo was intuitively led to rediscover these healing frequencies in the Book of Numbers (a book in the Old Testament), using a numerological technique to decipher the six repeating codes he found. The result was the rediscovery of the Solfeggio Frequencies.

Physicist, inventor, and electrical engineer Nikola Tesla once said, *"If you only knew the magnificence of the three, six and nine, then you would hold a key to the universe."* Interestingly, these three numbers form the root vibration of the six Solfeggio Frequencies.

These are the Solfeggio Frequencies:

1. UT 396 Hz: UTqueant laxis – liberation from guilt and fear.
2. RE 417 Hz: REsonare fibris - clears negativity and removes subconscious blockages.
3. MI 528 Hz: MIra gestorum - stimulates love, restores equilibrium, repairs DNA.
4. FA 639 Hz: FAmuli tuorum - strengthens relationships, family, and community unity.
5. SOL 741 Hz: SOLve polluti - physically cleanses the body from all types of toxins.
6. LA 852 Hz: LAbii reatum - awakening intuition and helps you return to spiritual balance.

These frequencies can be extremely beneficial for the human body and mind.

Fulvic minerals – Shilajit

I started integrating fulvic minerals into my life as I had been recognising for a while that soil standards, even organic, were significantly depleted. I do go through phases with it, sometimes it will be months where I don't take it and then I engage in a flurry of taking it because I am feeling the pull towards it, in particular during autumn and leading into winter months. Fulvic acid occurs naturally in all soils and research has revealed that it may bolster the defence of various health issues. It has been shown to fight inflammation and boost immune health added to water and taken a few times a day. Fulvic acid is also found in a product called shilajit, a tar-like sticky substance found in Himalayan mountain rocks - shilajit has been used in traditional eastern and ayurvedic medicine in India and Nepal for rejuvenating properties. It contains high amounts of fulvic acid, which in turn helps with inflammation.

Liver Detox - Milk Thistle

As I was working in the health field, I learnt that the liver had such a huge job to do and when I would sometimes feel run down, out of sync from teaching and working, I turned to milk thistle to support my liver to detoxify. This herbal tincture helped to cleanse and purify the liver, which in turn enhanced the absorption of food, nutrients, and vitamin and mineral supplements I was taking. Being the largest gland in the body and connected deeply to the skin, I would find that whatever was happening with my skin was a sign that my liver was needing some support. I went through a phase of dealing with pompholyx eczema between my fingers, appearing suddenly - very itchy watery blisters affecting the sides of fingers. This was so painful and inflamed and to me it was a sign that something was being released from my liver. On top of using homemade chamomile and extra virgin olive oil topically on the inflamed areas, I would detox with milk thistle.

The functions of the liver are (but not exclusive):

- Make bile - needed to digest fats.
- Keeps the blood clean and well-maintained.
- Help fight infections.
- Get rid of poisons.
- Stores energy in the form of glycogen.
- Makes and regulates many hormones, including sex hormones.
- Acts as a larder for e.g. vitamin B12, iron and fat soluble vitamin D.

Milk Thistle has a long history of traditional use and has been shown to support liver health and assist healthy digestive processes. I would always choose a company with ethical values and organic ingredients with no fillers. Usually, I would use the tincture instead of capsules, this is my preference.

EFT - Emotional Freedom Technique

EFT is a form of tapping, developed by Gary Craig, a civil engineer back in 1995, although there are many similar kinds of 'tapping' practices. I return to his original teaching every time on the subject. Once learned, it is a self-healing tool that can be incredibly helpful in day-to-day life. It provides a sequence and a means of balancing the energy system, allowing the body's own system to re-align itself by tapping the meridians as outlined by traditional Chinese medicine, a little like acupuncture only this time with hands. The aim is to clear negative emotions and associated physical or psychological manifestations and create space between the emotional 'charge' and the body response. EFT takes a few minutes to learn but isn't a one-minute wonder, it is something that can build over days and time.

I have turned to EFT many times and have found it to be really helpful in soothing my emotional self. In particular, Brad Yates on YouTube has a large variety of videos that you can follow along, one particular one I really like is 'Raise your Vibration'.

Kinesiology - Muscle Testing

After working in further and higher education, I found my whole energy system was taking a hit. This was a very challenging and stressful profession to enter - teaching! I didn't think it through very well, although I had always been interested in education and training, it was a very depleting profession to enter. As I was now in a more balanced state of health, I wanted to ensure I could deal with all that was being sent my way, preparing and planning lessons, resources, the actual art of teaching and presenting, and managing all that life offered; I was also stepping into married life. Kinesiology was where I turned to help me to maintain balance with my professional life. This holistic practice aims to restore balance to the whole person through promoting the self-healing capacity. It is a non-invasive holistic energy therapy that combines ancient Chinese medicine principles with muscle monitoring techniques, using the body as a diagnostic tool to explore health status. The premise is that any problems that arise will be seen in the energy system before appearing in the body. I used to go to a kinesiologist who would muscle test me, not for food this time but for questions relating to self-care, managing my time, workload and relationships to name but a few.

Flotation - Salt Baths

I went for my first float as I was beginning to see changes in the early 90s. I had been ill for about four years, and my friend suggested it as a new floatation centre had opened. It was a very new concept and we booked an introductory session. This was a whole new experience, I absolutely loved it; not long after this centre opened, one appeared nearer to where I lived.

I didn't realise at the time the benefits of floating, but I soon discovered with more research that it has been scientifically proven to increase mental and physical wellbeing in just the hour it takes to settle into a float. It can alleviate aches and pains in the body and encourage a better night's sleep. Due to the fact that external stimulus is shut off, the body can truly relax, in a weightless environment. It can also help to soothe stresses and strains of the mind.

I later turned to Epsom salt baths. A tried and tested home remedy, Epsom Salts have long been used as a therapeutic alternative for a range of ailments as well as to help the body recover after sport and exercise. For example:

- Easing strains and relaxing tired, stiff or aching muscles.
- Relieves pain and muscle cramps. Promotes sleep and stress reduction.
- Soothes nervous and digestive systems. Helps to eliminate toxins from the body.

Morning pages - The Artist's Way

The morning pages are three pages of long hand stream of consciousness writing done first thing in the morning. They were first outlined in The Artist's Way by Julia Cameron, I first came across this book around 1997, which was transformational. It was a twelve-week programme to connect or reconnect to the creative artist within each and every one of us, and there were approaches to integrate into one's day, the morning pages being one of them.

> "*There is no wrong way to do Morning Pages– they are not high art. They are not even writing. They are about anything and everything that crosses your mind – and they are for your eyes only. Morning Pages provoke, clarify, comfort, cajole, prioritise and synchronise the day at hand. Do not overthink Morning Pages: just put three pages of anything on the page...and then do three more pages tomorrow.*" Julia Cameron

I began with pads of A4 lined paper, which I kept to the side of my bed. I began to write and write and write - at first there was a lot of '*I have no idea what I'm supposed to write, why am I doing this*' or, '*I better get dressed and out of bed, what do I need today?* and then after writing a whole load of this something flipped. I would begin to flow, so I let the words take off. What used to happen were creative splurges, I may write a poem, or have an epiphany about a specific problem that needed sorting. This is one of the non-negotiables of The Artist's Way and there are twelve weeks to work through, a book I would highly recommend.

Gratitudes

It was in 1998 that I first read Simple Abundance by Sarah Ban Breathnach. This book offered 365 days of comfort and joy and I used to read one every day and decided there and then I would begin to write a gratitude list every evening at the end of my day. I would find a lovely journal that would give me a buzz when I opened it (another notebook Julia!) and write five things I was grateful for at the end of that day. These may range from going out for lunch with my lovely Mum, a comfy bed and pillows, the sun shining, some funny antics from my dogs, Lucy, Luna, Honey, or Pudding the Cat, the time I spent chatting to my neighbour, seeing the smile from my nieces or long deep chats with those close to me. It got me into a flow of seeing what was around me, in a much more present way, and this connected me to attracting uplifting energy. Sarah Ban Breathnach recognised how gratitude cultivated healing, joy, authenticity, balance and wholeness. I found this really helped me to flip my days before going to bed at night, by sending uplifting messages to my subconscious mind for sleep. Messages that would marinate through the night.

The Honeyscrub

Once I decided to cut out chemicals in cosmetics and cleaning products, I wanted to make my own. In the very early days, I bought a book by Liz Earle called Natural Beauty. At that time, she was a health journalist for GMTV (Good Morning Television in the UK) before she created her naturally active skincare range and long before she sold out to L'Oréal. She profiled how to make different types of products for cleansing, toning and moisturising using simple ingredients.

I have gone through phases of creating my skin care but now I use a cleanser, washed off with a hot face cloth, spritzed with pure organic rose water and moisturised with a either 100% organic rosehip oil, sweet almond oil, carrot oil, vitamin E oil I choose depending on my mood. I have also in the past used Tropic, which is a beautiful plant-based brand. The less ingredients, the better for me.

One of my delights is a body exfoliator I called The Honeyscrub. This has become a ritual for me once a month, it is better than any exfoliator I have used previously and smells lush on its own without any essential oils because of the honey. However, you don't have to use honey if you're plant-based; you could use a little bit of maple syrup. However, if you do, try to find a local organic honey.

Mix the following ingredients in a small cereal bowl until you have a nice consistency, not runny or too thick. Coarse or fine salt (depends on how rough/smooth you want it).

- Honey.
- Porridge oats / milled.
- Extra Virgin Olive Oil (EVOO).
- Celtic salt

This is for the body, so if you're making it for your face, you'll need a gentler mix: use fine salt, honey, fine oats, plus sweet almond oil, maybe organic aloe vera gel.

In the shower and without turning it on yet, gently begin to scoop up small handfuls; you may find it flies around, so don't use too much at once. Once you're scrubbed, turn the shower on and wash off, your skin will adore it and you'll smell divine and yummy.

These are back to basics; I know your body will thank you for taking it back to the foundation level and using nature's products. Adding synthetic chemicals can often have such a huge impact. My Mum advocated soap and water for washing her face and cleaning her body, she had great skin and hands up to her older years. I also use homemade organic soap and a face-cloth for washing my body and hands. Less chemical intervention, less intrusion, less waste - your immune system will thank you for it.

Belly Dancing - Dance like No One is Watching

I first went to belly dancing while working in further education as a lecturer and was hooked. The combination of the beat of the Middle Eastern vibe and the movement of my body, I couldn't get over how beautiful it felt. I had spent over a decade feeling sore and restricted in movement, tired and depleted, yet here I was, twelve years later, feeling like I had found my beat again. It was momentous. I threw myself into belly dancing. I went every week, I bought the music, I went to concerts, (thank you, Natacha Atlas.) I felt like I was a woman again. I bought belly dancing belts to wrap around my hips; the sound was hypnotic, I danced like no one was watching (PS they weren't). I adored it. For me at that moment, I felt like I had found my way. I would flit in and out of this dancing, but if ever there is a time when by Natacha Atlas comes on to my playlist, you can find me shimmying my hips in the figure eight and waving my hands in the air!

Now this may not be for all of you, but the idea here is to dance like nobody's watching, gather your music playlist, and find all the songs that get you clicking your fingers and vibing high. Dance and know that you're raising your vibration. For so many years, I just couldn't find the energy to boogie; it was wonderful when I could.

Feng Shui - the Art of Placement

From my early years in primary school, I intuitively used to rearrange my bedroom. Every six months I would change around my bed from one wall to the next, there weren't many options due to alcoves and shelving, but little Julia wanted a different perspective out the window, so you would often find her upstairs after school, shifting things round, tidying drawers and clearing out clutter. Little did I know that this was an aspect of feng shui which I discovered many years later.

Feng shui is a system for arranging your surroundings in harmony and balance with the natural world around you. Who knew that's what I was doing?!

This was about turning my attention to my space around me and changing it, reorganising furniture, tidying dark corners that were full of 'stuff,' clearing packed drawers, reviewing what was hanging around and what I was hanging on to, hidden. It is also related to clothing, what did I not wear, and what could I share. This wasn't something I did in the midst of ill health, but it has always been a place to turn to when I am or have been feeling like I wanted to shift gears. It was where I turned to when my health began to stabilise. My question to you is what are you hanging on to, what needs releasing, where is there clutter, what are you hoarding? Clearing our environments and being in harmony with the flow of rooms and directions can often be a trigger for other light bulb moments. This takes us to living more minimally and simply with less stuff and things.

Going into feng shui in more detail you will discover the bagua, a map of placement for different areas of our life.

Massage - Muscles Remember

As I have written earlier, when I was in the throes of ME, massage was too depleting for my body. I didn't go back to this for a decade but as I began working in education, every now and again, I would step back into the world of massage, discovering what the beautiful process of deep tissue Swedish massage, or hot stone was for my body, mind and soul. I have tried a variety of different types of massage and in further research I found that massage can relieve the body of its stored trauma, which is held within the fascia, muscles, tendons, even cells; therefore, without having to talk about any issues at hand, massage can be an additional approach to releasing.

There was always a chance it would send me into a spiral of feeling very tired again, although, I knew this wouldn't last, I would take the nudge and go to rest. On occasions I would feel energised and other times, I may experience a 'healing crisis' showing up with a runny nose, a headache, or feeling sore; this was my body's way of detoxing. I never saw this as a negative situation, it was a clearing of stuck energy.

I have often said that if doctors would give prescriptions for weekly massages in lieu of written prescriptions for antidepressants, they would discover a much happier and healthier patient quota, because the power of touch and massage can work wonders for mental, physical, emotional and spiritual health.

ReBalancing Toolkit

Now you have read through all the book and jotted down any notes. Do you have somewhere you'd like to begin? Is there a particular Way pulling you? Would you like to add some different ideas to the Ways? Have you ticked off some already because they are familiar? Which is Your Way? It's over to you, this is the where you create your own ReBalancing Toolkit. Let's revisit them.

BO-NO-SO-CO-CRE-MO

The First Way: BOOST

1. **Vitamins and Minerals** *Pause*: Supplement Me
2. **Bye Bye Sugar** *Pause*: You're Sweet Enough
3. **Probiotic Possibilities** *Pause*: Your Insides Guide
4. **Echinacea** *Pause*: Blooming Daisy
5. **Organic and Seasonal** *Pause*: F&V Organically

The Second Way : NOURISH

1. **Food Combining** *Pause*: Release the Grain
2. **Hydration** *Pause*: Water In, Water Out
3. **Chemical Clear Out** *Pause*: The Chemical Bothers
4. **Earthing** *Pause*: Ground Yourself
5. **Journalling** *Pause*: Write Your Inside Out

The Third Way: SUPPORT

1. **Aromatherapy** *Pause*: Essential Smells
2. **Reflexology** *Pause*: Feet Know
3. **Bach Flower Remedies** *Pause*: Get Bach
4. **Counselling** *Pause*: Voice it
5. **Reiki** *Pause*: Radiant Energy

The Fourth Way : COCOON

1. **Ditch the News** *Pause*: Release the Drip
2. **Peace and Quiet** *Pause*: The Magic Chair
3. **No Means No** *Pause*: Know your Compass
4. **Bedtime Ritual** *Pause*: Flow to Sleep
5. **Electronics EMF** *Pause*: Tech Fast

The Fifth Way : CREATE

1. **Shift the Focus** *Pause*: Follow the Cues
2. **Vision On** *Pause*: Imagining You
3. **Colour Spectrum** *Pause*: Colouring In
4. **Soothing Deck** *Pause*: Cards Lift Up
5. **Elevate your Vibe** *Pause*: Film Joy

The Sixth Way : MOVE

1. **Affirm Up** *Pause*: Flip the Lines
2. **Calm your Nerves** *Pause*: Box Breathing
3. **Feel the Sphere** *Pause*: The Ball of Chi
4. **Shake it Out** *Pause*: Get ChiQi
5. **Letter- it Go** *Pause*: Dear Dot Dot Dot

You may want to note below any ideas that have popped up as you revisit The Ways, practitioners you already know who can help, books you have on your bookshelf to read, friends, colleagues who may help you, plus now you're nearly at the end, you may want to research further to find a practitioner to help and support you.

Conclusion

We have reached the end. Time to breathe and take this all in.

I know there has been a great deal to digest throughout these pages and I am trusting that you will gravitate to the approaches that you are feeling called to explore. This is the book that I wished I had to read when I was ill thirty-six years ago. Sharing my Six Ways with you has been an introduction into rebooting and recalibrating your whole body and mind; if there is anywhere you are particularly drawn to, go there first. Take it in stages, this isn't a place where you have to rush or push. Consider what you're resonating towards and try this for a few weeks or months, see the effect, keep a notebook so you can record your feelings and notice changes to physiological responses in your body and changes in symptoms.

Throughout these pages, my intention has been for you to create your own ReBalancing Toolkit for your day-to-day life. Think of this as a box, in it are the signposts; Boost, Nourish, Support, Cocoon, Create, Move, within them choose your

Way Points. Ask yourself '*what do I need today, what is calling me*? Pick the one that works for you, start with one, two or three approaches. You'll find you begin to add more and more of your own as you investigate and research further, as you continue on the boomerang's flight path.

Be conscious of the signposts - do you need a boost, what are you consuming both internally and externally, what is nourishing you? What support are you seeking, you can't do this all by yourself, you need a team of practitioners and therapists around you. How are you breathing? Are you taking time out to meditate and have some P&Q? What are you creating in your day, is there something missing? Can you shift the focus and generate a different mindset? Where is the movement, either internally or externally depending on your starting point. What kind of movement does your body need?

Feel your way through this, let go of analytical thought, go back to your gut instinct, get in touch with your heart. Your intuition knows.

You have to get quiet in order to hear the messages that your body and your higher self is nudging you towards.

Afterword by Sheila Dolowitch

There have been many books written about Myalgic Encephalomyelitis (ME). Now it is a recognised illness, there is more knowledge than ever before with specific guidelines that professionals adhere to. Yet, this appalling illness has so many different symptoms that it proves to be a challenge. Each individual needs to be treated holistically.

My dear daughter Julia is one of the fortunate few who has recovered. My family and I sincerely thank the specialists, doctors and complementary practitioners who tried to make a difference for her, especially the ones who believed her and also diagnosed that it was indeed ME. These people were very few and far between when this was happening to Julia at the beginning of 1990. It was hard to find out who they were and even harder to find where they were.

In the early years of this ill health, we discovered her immune system was not working correctly; hence, we were advised to embark upon a stringent vitamin and mineral programme. Back then, it was the first place to start; there was no definite idea at that time of what to do because there was no directive from anyone.

Not only did Julia struggle to overcome all that invaded her body with such ferocity, but so did I. How did we cope when nobody believed us? How did we get through together? It was with lots of perseverance, humour and in harmony.

We tried most things to alleviate her awful symptoms.

I recall crying to close friends, asking, "*what will she do if she does ever get better? She is just starting out; what will her life be like?*"

They replied, "*let her get better first and then she will find her feet.*"

Looking back now, as I write from 2005, I had heard of Myalgic Encephalomyelitis known as ME. But honestly, I didn't want to admit it at that early stage, in case everyone thought I was deranged. The media were busy calling it 'Yuppie Flu' and the more I listened to the radio or read the relevant newspaper reports, the more it gave me grave cause for concern.

An acquaintance had a daughter who had been ill with ME for several years. I met her one day and she told me about her.

"*Are you sure Julia does not have ME?*" she asked me.

She then proceeded to tell me the symptoms to look for and described exactly what Julia was going through: extreme tiredness and fatigue, no energy to move, muscle aching, cold extremities, dizziness, sore throat, swollen glands, and as I listened to her my heart sank lower and lower.

"*That is exactly what I am worried about,*" I told her.

In those very early weeks, I made an appointment with one of the doctors that I used to see. I had known my doctor for many years and wanted to ask him about ME. As I began telling him about Julia and her symptoms, he looked at me and said, "*Oh, it's fashionable.*" He dismissed the whole idea. I tried to persevere, but he took no notice. This intolerable situation could not go on without professional help, so I went to the library to see what I could find out about ME but there was nothing to be found. Very odd. Surely someone knew enough to write about it but obviously not.

We read in a newspaper that a gastroenterologist in Rodney Street, Liverpool, was specialising in ME. We made an appointment via Julia's GP, Dr Griffiths, and took her to see him. He examined Julia and spoke with her at length. After listening to her, he was very helpful and concluded that she had post-viral fatigue syndrome and could possibly be the beginnings of ME.

He said that Julia would not be able to go back to work for at least six months, so when we got back home after much discussion with each other and with Dr Griffiths, she telephoned her employer in Manchester and told him the outcome. He said he would put one month's money into her account and wished her well.

In March, I went to her flat in Manchester, packed my car with all her belongings and came home. Driving home, I felt very, very sad. The nauseating feeling that this was the end of the beginning or the beginning of the end would not go away. My mind was in turmoil and I kept thinking about what would happen to Julia now. How will she get over this debilitating illness? Worse yet, will she ever get better and back to normal?

I drove into the next service station, parked the car and sat crying my heart out. I sobbed for so long that I lost track of time, but I eventually pulled myself together, bought a cup of strong coffee and drove home. Some things one can forget but that incident will stay in my memory forever.

I was in despair throughout the first three years of Julia's illness. My mission was to bring her some relief and find a way through, but nothing seemed to work.

What impressed me was her attitude. She never once complained, never felt sorry for herself and always said that when she got better, she would know the reason for the illness. She felt there would be an explanation for it all.

What an attitude for someone so young.

Watching a loved one going through any illness is a trying experience, as the constant helplessness of being unable to improve things is intolerable. Desiring to do something practical is paramount. I did not feel normal, caring for Julia was taking up my time and my life, but I wouldn't change a thing.

I clearly remember my dreams in different formats that constantly troubled me. They always took place in a railway station and Julia was lying on the tracks but could not get up and I could not lift her up. People stood by and looked down on her but just stared at her and did not try to assist me. That was the dream that took place two or three times each week. I wasn't frightened of it and knew that it was me trying to free Julia from her illness.

There was no let-up in caring; it was not just a daytime duty but twenty-four hours attention, and it was love and hopelessness at the awful situation and the intense desire to take the ME away from my dear youngest daughter.

I constantly worried that ME would never leave and Julia would be ill for the rest of her life. As much as I tried to talk sense to myself, I kept getting the idea that this was indeed for life.

The emotional burden complicated this practical burden. All we, and every sufferer and carer, wants is a speedy diagnosis but we seemed to come across a stonewall whichever way we turned. If only the medical profession could have been more positive, but I suppose they were early days. I did not care about 'early days'; I just wanted Julia to be healed but nobody seemed to take ME seriously.

I am writing this in 2005 and ME is taken more seriously.

Julia's ME was attributed to an initial virus, exacerbated by a weakened immune system, antibiotic overuse and candidiasis - in those early days of her tonsillitis, she almost lived on them. Nowadays, doctors are more aware of prescribing them, which is absolutely correct, and people are more mindful. The damage they can cause outweighs the good they do as they were too often handed out like sweets.

Now Julia is well again. I wonder how I coped, but I did; while the problem was ongoing, I just accepted the circumstances and got on with life. However, now that I think of my uncontrollable situation, I am still amazed at my strength. How I got through it, I don't really know; all I wanted to do was to make Julia better and that was the main aim of my life. I have said it before, It was a natural pull and I have no regrets. Friends asked me how I managed and I replied that I am not sure, but whatever predicaments happen in families, they need to be met head-on. No family gets away with problems, however small or big, they just have to be handled in the best possible way.

One doesn't have time to think about how to cope; one gets on with whatever one is presented with. That sounds hard and cold-hearted but that is life. No books tell you how to manage; you use common sense and muddle through. The carer always takes the brunt of the problem as they try to take the pain away from their loved one. They also are the ones who have to explain about the ailment and often take disparaging comments from people.

After she finally got the help she needed from the consultants Dr Downing and Dr Collins. Julia began her anti-candida way of eating, plus all the vitamin and mineral supplements, IV drips and the support she sought from the complementary therapists; I could see Julia taking a turn for the better. We were all jubilant and thought this could be the beginning of the end. I kept telling myself not to be too complacent, but inside, I could not help feeling a little excited.

Apart from my family, I got very little support except from a few personal loyal friends who listened and tried to give me advice on how to deal with it. I was very grateful for them as they propped me up. I tried very hard not to bore them with my feelings but it came out because it had to and they were my help. They did not know much about ME, but they listened to me.

So many people do not get over ME; they are tragically afflicted for life. Thankfully Julia was on the right path and I was very happy to take a back seat. Her precious years can never be replaced, however hard one may try and I have to be so thankful that she found her way through.

People still ask me how she is and now, in 2005, I am delighted to inform them that "*Julia is very well, thank you.*"

I have been trying to think of how to put into words how I feel and the other day, I came across a small card with very special words that validated exactly how I feel in my heart.

I remember looking at you when you were a child wondering what your future would hold.
I wanted to shelter you from unhappiness and surround you only with wonderful things.
I realise now that I could not have done this, for in order to appreciate happiness you had to experience disappointment.
To enjoy success you had to have some failure.
To feel true love someone had to break your heart.
I couldn't protect you but I wanted you to know I was with you every step of the way.
When I look at you now and see the woman that has emerged from within I could not be more proud.

We are so thankful for her good health now. I love you darling Julia. I am always here for you and will watch over you forever.

Sheila Dolowitch
Written in 2005.

Mum, reading your words from 2005, now the afterword of my book, is all the more poignant as you're no longer here. I know you would be steeped in joy at this being published.

This book has been waiting in the wings. I began it many years ago; we would talk about it often back in the day. Now and then, I would have more lightbulb moments and spend time writing on it. Then a curve ball would hit and I'd take a step back.

After your passing, I would hear the whispers, usually in the very early hours of the morning, '*write, Julia, write*,' so I turned to the written word again and opened the text I had begun years earlier.

I feel you know that this is happening and you're watching over me.

Mum, thank you for being my 'strength extraordinaire.' You were an incredible force.

Your huge protective spirit, unstoppable determination to help, support and find answers, massive amounts of love and care, and an abundance of humour pulled us through the dark times.

With love, always

Your daughter Julia

Postscript

The Way of the Boomerang is a way of life for me, it has become more profound as I moved through bereavement. I revisited the original Ways and added new ones to help me heal and deal. It's not about getting it right all the time or being perfect in any given approach, these are gentle ways to rebalance.

I do not have it all sorted, am by no means perfect, and am continuously a 'being in progress', what I know for sure is that I am an avid health researcher and investigator, I have to explore from my own perspective, assess, review, and pause to reflect.

What grabs my attention these days is the power of healing through sound, hertz frequencies and scalar energy. When exploring these modalities and techniques you discover they have been around for a very long time but have been removed and repressed from western medical systems, although they are beginning to be revealed, once again. During the last couple of years, I have embarked upon more supportive healing, for example sound technology and harmonics, infrared sauna, halotherapy (salt) and acupuncture. Whilst doing so engaging with other practitioners, authors, experts in their holistic fields of medicine, I uncover yet again that many dis-eases and dis-orders are as a consequence of our environment and not because of our genetics. Thanks to Dr Bruce Lipton founder of epigenetics, whom I first saw speak in Albuquerque, New Mexico in 2004 at the 6th International Conference on Science and Consciousness, I continue to see the deep connection twenty years later.

In my daily life, I weave all these new unfolding discoveries into The Six Ways; **Boost, Nourish, Support, Cocoon, Create, Move.** I don't do everything all the time, but I know what's in my ReBalancing Toolkit and where I need to turn to develop my own prescription when curve balls hit or when I'm dealing with something.

My attention is now focused exploring and experiencing new approaches for the future of our health and wellbeing and that of the earth and all this realm in which we reside, all earthlings, on two legs, four, with wings, or fins. I have seen a huge re-emergence in energy medicine, and the use of sound technologies and frequencies; this is where I keep my eyes peeled. Below I have highlighted some examples I follow and continue to research.

Rife Frequencies

Dr Royal Raymond Rife in the early 1930's discovered that all medical conditions have an electro-magnetic frequency and developed the Rife machine which worked by finding the frequency of the condition in the body and an impulse of the same frequency was then used to kill or dis-able diseased cells. There is a significant amount of information around the Rife machine, it has been degraded and dismissed, however, keep watching because the FDA (Food and Drug Administration) has recently approved a $12,000 cancer treatment that uses sound waves to disintegrate tumours as a painless alternative to radiation and chemotherapy. This is primarily used in liver tumours and has been developed by company called Histo-Sonics founded in 2009. The technique is called histotripsy and generates exploding bubbles to kill tumours.

www.rife.org

The Energy Enhancement System

The EE system generates multiple bio-active life enhancing energy fields, including "scalar waves" which can allow cell regeneration, improve immune function, provide relief from pain, detoxify the body, elevate moods, and assist in balancing right and left hemispheres of the brain to increase energy levels.

Developed over 20 years ago by Dr. Sandra Rose Michael, Ph.D, DNM, DCSJl, it uses custom-installed computers to generate morphogenic energy fields that can promote healing. The EESystem has been recognised at dozens of medical, scientific and professional conferences around the world. These systems have been installed internationally to promote wellness, healing, relaxation, purification and rejuvenation. This is very much one to watch. There are a number of EE systems in the UK find the one nearest to you. I can recommend highly The Zenergy Centre in Cleckheaton, West Yorkshire

www.thezenergycentre.co.uk

www.eesystem.com/center-locator

The Harmonic Egg

The Harmonic Egg invented by Gail Lynn is new to the UK from the USA having has been here for about three years. It is a sound and light frequency chamber that envelops the body once you are immersed inside to create an environment that allows the body to heal from many ailments. When you are comfortably reclined on a zero-gravity chair, light frequency, vibration and sound create a blend of energy to stimulate one's autonomic system to reorganise and promote homeostasis (balance) back into the body. Scientific contributions from neuroscience, molecular biology, and physics are now actively supporting energy or "frequency medicine" as it is referred to, as a legitimate alternative to heal the body. This treatment is risk free, repeatable and has no side effects. There is only one in the UK, based in Suffolk with plans for more prototypes soon.

www.harmoniceggheling.co.uk

Hyperbaric Oxygen Chamber (HBOT)

During hyperbaric oxygen therapy, pure oxygen is delivered to the lungs under increased atmospheric pressure in a hyperbaric chamber. The extra oxygen saturates the red blood cells and is carried through the blood plasma delivering this to all tissues in the body; stimulating cell growth and repairs damage to cells and organs. It can help with relief in symptoms from post viral fatigue syndrome, low energy, neuro inflammation, though it is not a medical aid. It is also one to watch. Search for HBOT one recommendation is Your Health Bank.

www.yourhealthbank.co.uk

Photobiomodulation

According to Dr Damien Downing, 'Photo-bio-modulation – light (photo) changing (modulating) life processes (bio). It used to be called LLLT - Low Level Laser Therapy - but now more and more is being done with more ordinary LED lights.'

What health issues is light good for? He writes "just about everything, this is a list of ailments that I could find at least some evidence for benefits."

- Inflammation - possibly all forms
- Infections - probably all micro-organisms (bacteria, fungi, viruses, parasites like malaria)
- Fatigue - possibly whatever the cause
- Fibromyalgia
- Oedema and swelling
- Mucositis
- Physical and ischaemic injury
- Chronic pain
- Wound healing
- Toxic burden
- Brain trauma
- Neurodegenerative - Parkinson's, Alzheimer's
- Autoimmune disease - Alopecia, Hashimoto's, MS
- Ageing (learning, attention, memory, cognitive decline)
- Type 2 diabetes
- Depression & anxiety
- Athletic performance enhancement

Treatment can be through intravenous, transdermal, transcranial, interstitial, intranasal, oral.

www.drdamiendowning.com

Infra Red

The infrared sauna experience is different from traditional sauna, it helps to rebalance deep from inside the cell. The infrared light penetrates directly to the core increasing the body temperature by 3° causing a false 'fever' effect, which stimulates immune function and makes the body less habitable for pathogens. 20% detoxification is achieved as opposed to 3% in traditional saunas. Heavy metals, toxins and stagnant hormones are eliminated from the body enabling cells to function more efficiently. Health benefits include improving circulation, releasing toxins, lowers blood pressure, relieves aches and pains, reduces fatigue, decreases cortisol (stress hormone), increases deep sleep. This again is not a medical device but one to watch and explore. You can find infrared saunas now throughout the UK.

It has been nearly two years since I dedicated myself to writing The Way of the Boomerang. Revisiting my story, stepping back into that time of Julia in her twenties, incapacitated, dis-abled and with her life on hold, I saw a young woman who courageously moved through the tunnel to the other side.

In writing this book, I re-examined how I got through back then, the steps I took, the learning I gleaned, all the support and help I received, not only from consultants and practitioners but from Mum, family and close friends around me. After my health was impacted from significant losses, The Way of the Boomerang began to help me once again.

I found myself re-turning to the fundamental ways that refuelled my tank. I have tapped back into approaches to stay afloat. I ebb and flow, I move up and down, I am a work in progress.

Writing this book and the publishing journey has been a huge learning curve. I have found a renewed sense of purpose rebuilding my holistic health practice; meeting and supporting new clients has spurred me on. I can dream and imagine again, I can give back and support those around me.

It is my honour and privilege to bring this book to light. I sincerely hope you find a spark within these pages, helping you, your clients, and those you care about on your boomerang journey.

Julia

with the canine crew

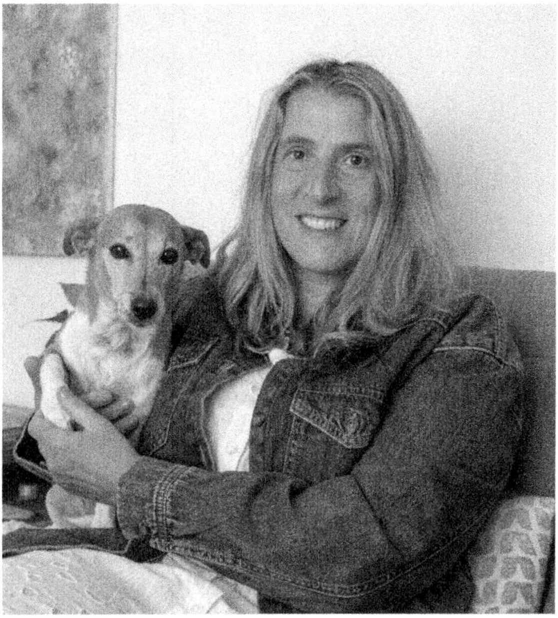

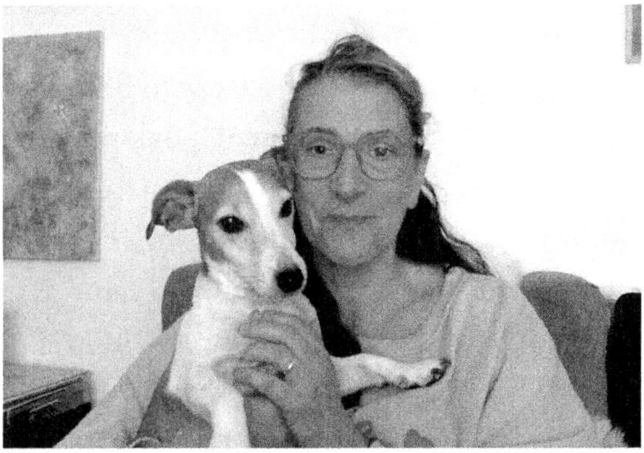

Evidence

When I began my quest to heal ME as a young 21-year-old, I was being drawn to different approaches based on all I was experiencing and reading. One book led to another, one practitioner to the next. Thirty-six years on, the methods that I have shared are much more in the medical and wellness arena; many of them may not be surprising to you now, yet back then, it was unusual and very quacky to be doing some of the things I was doing. They were often 'pooh-poohed' or sniggered at because I was stepping out of the usual comfort zone.

In writing The Way of the Boomerang, I decided to go further still and I found evidence relating to some, if not most of the Way Points, thereby highlighting how things that were once considered fringe, quirky or sniffed at, are validated today. Many of the methods I explored have since gained the backing of scientific research. I am not incorporating the following studies and articles to "prove" the efficacy of my chosen methods, rather so that you can begin to investigate more deeply should you wish to explore further. I hope that this consequently helps to combine my experiential wisdom with scientific integrity and therefore broaden the scope of what you see as possible.

Please visit www.aepress.co.uk to find all the active links listed, if you are reading the printed book.

BOOST
Vitamins and Minerals

Vitamin C

Hemilä, H. Vitamin C and Infections. *Nutrients.* 2017, 9, 339. https://doi.org/10.3390/nu9040339

Vitamin C: IV Drips

Huang L, Wang L, Tan J, Liu H, Ni Y. High-dose vitamin C intravenous infusion in the treatment of patients with COVID-19: A protocol for systematic review and meta-analysis. *Medicine (Baltimore).* 2021 May 14;100(19):e25876. https://dio.org/10.1097/MD.0000000000025876. PMID: 34106642; PMCID: PMC8133047. https://bit.ly/highdosevitamincintravenousinfusion

Vitamin D

McCullough PJ, Lehrer DS, Amend J. Daily oral dosing of vitamin D3 using 5000 TO 50,000 international units a day in long-term hospitalized patients: Insights from a seven year experience. *The Journal of Steroid Biochemistry and Molecular Biology.* 2019 May;189:228-239. https://doi.org/10.1016/j.jsbmb.2018.12.010

Wimalawansa, S.J. Physiological Basis for Using Vitamin D to Improve Health. *Biomedicines* 2023,11, 1542. https://doi.org/10.3390/biomedicines11061542

Sugar

Gillespie, Kerri M., Kemps Eva, White, Melanie J, and Bartlett Selena E. The Impact of Free Sugar on Human Health — A Narrative Review. 2023 *Nutrients* 15, no. 4: 889. https://doi.org/10.3390/nu15040889

Jawhara, Samir. Healthy Diet and Lifestyle Improve the Gut Microbiota and Help Combat Fungal Infection. *Microorganisms*11, 2023. no. 6: 1556. https://doi.org/10.3390/microorganisms11061556

Probiotics

Kechagia M, Basoulis D, Konstantopoulou S, Dimitriadi D, Gyftopoulou K, Skarmoutsou N, Fakiri EM. Health Benefits of Probiotics: A Review. *ISRN Nutr.* 2013 Jan 2;2013:481651. PMID: 24959545; PMCID: PMC4045285 https://doi.org/10.5402/2013/481651

Maftei, Nicoleta-Maricica, Cosmin Raducu Raileanu, Alexia Anastasia Balta, Lenuta Ambrose, Monica Boev, Denisa Batîr Marin, and Elena Lacramioara Lisa. The Potential Impact of Probiotics on Human Health: An Update on Their Health-Promoting Properties. 2024 *Microorganisms* 12, no. 2: 234. https://doi.org/10.3390/microorganisms12020234

Echinacea

Sachin A Shah PharmD, Stephen Sander PharmD, C Michael White PharmD, Mike Rinaldi PharmD, Dr Craig I Coleman PharmD Evaluation of echinacea for the prevention and treatment of the common cold: a meta-analysis Lancet. *Infectious Diseases* 2007;7:473-80 https://doi.org/10.1016/S1473-3099(07)70160-3 https://bit.ly/thelancetevaluationofechinacea

Organic and Seasonal

Ajmer Singh Grewal, Ashish Singla, Pradeep Kamboj, Jagdeep Singh Dua Pesticide Residues in Food Grains, Vegetables and Fruits: A Hazard to Human Health Publish Date. 2017-03-20 *Journal of Medicinal Chemistry and Toxicology* https://www.ommegaonline.org/article-details/Pesticide-Residues-in-Food-Grains-Vegetables-and-Fruits-A-Hazard-to-Human-Health/1355#REFERENCES

Rosca M., Cozma, P. and Hlihor, R.M., Environmental and human impacts of the toxic pesticides use in agriculture: a review. *Proc. Rom. Acad.*, Series B, 2023, 25(3), p. 185–191 https://acad.ro/sectii2002/proceedingsChemistry/doc2023-3/Art4MihaelaRosca.pdf

NOURISH
Food Combining

Dasriya, V.L., Samtiya, M., Ranveer, S., Dhillon, H.S., Devi, N., Sharma, V., Nikam, P., Puniya, M., Chaudhary, P., Chaudhary, V., Behare, P.V., Dhewa, T., Vemuri, R., Raposo, A., Puniya, D.V., Khedkar, G.D., Vishweswaraiah, R.H., Vij, S., Alarifi, S.N., Han, H. and Puniya, A.K. Modulation of gut-microbiota through probiotics and dietary interventions to improve host health. 2024 *Journal of Science and Food Agriculture* published by John Wiley & Sons Ltd on behalf of Society of Chemical Industry. https://doi.org/10.1002/jsfa.13370

Hydration

Maureen Twiddy, Jeanette M. Rotchell Evangelos Danopoulos Microplastic contamination of drinking water: A systematic review. Published: July 31, 2020 https://doi.org/10.1371/journal.pone.0236838 *Plos One*: https://dx.plos.org/10.1371/journal.pone.0236838

Wee, S.Y., Aris, A.Z., Yusoff, F.M. et al. Occurrence of multiclass endocrine disrupting compounds in a drinking water supply system and associated risks. *Sci Rep 10*, 17755 (2020). https://doi.org/10.1038/s41598-020-74061-5

Li Lin1 Haoran Yang1 Xiaocang Xu2 Front. Effects of Water Pollution on Human Health and Disease Heterogeneity: A Review. *Environ. Sci., Sec. Water and Wastewater Management* 30 June 2022 Volume 10 – 2022 https://doi.org/10.3389/fenvs.2022.880246 https://www.frontiersin.org/articles/10.3389/fenvs.2022.880246/full

Chemical Clear Out

Panico A, Serio F, Bagordo F, Grassi T, Idolo A, DE Giorgi M, Guido M, Congedo M, DE Donno A. Skin safety and health prevention: an overview of chemicals in cosmetic products. *J Prev Med Hyg*. 2019 Mar 29;60(1):E50-E57. https://doi.org/10.15167/2421-4248/jpmh2019.60.1.1080

Radin D, Hayssen G, Emoto M, Kizu T. Double-blind test of the effects of distant intention on water crystal formation. *Explore (NY).* 2006 Sep-Oct; 2(5):408-11. https://doi.org/10.1016/j.explore.2006.06.004 PMID: 16979104. https://waterjournal.org

Earthing

Oschman JL, Chevalier G, Brown R. The effects of grounding (earthing) on inflammation, the immune response, wound healing, and prevention and treatment of chronic inflammatory and autoimmune diseases. *J Inflamm Res.* 2015 Mar 24;8:83-96. https://doi.org/10.2147/JIR.S69656. PMID: 25848315; PMCID: PMC4378297. https://www.ncbi.nlm.nih.gov/pmc/articles/PMC4378297/

Journalling

Jeremy Sutton PhD 5 Benefits of Journaling for Mental Health. *Positive Psychology* 14 May 2018 modified 4 October 2023 https://positivepsychology.com/benefits-of-journaling

Reflection App Top Evidence-Based Benefits of Journaling for Mental Health. December 27, 2022 https://www.reflection.app/blog/benefits-of-journaling

Baikie KA, Wilhelm K. Emotional and physical health benefits of expressive writing. *Advances in Psychiatric Treatment.* 2005;11(5):338-346. https://doi.org/10.1192/apt.11.5.338

Peng, H., Ma, J., Hu, J., & Gan, Y. (2024). Association of daily stress with daily anxiety and depression: Roles of self-affirmation and positive attention bias. *European Journal of Health Psychology*, 31(1), 16–27. https://doi.org/10.1027/2512-8442/a000140

SUPPORT

Aromatherapy

Thangaleela, Subramanian, Bhagavathi Sundaram Sivamaruthi, Periyanaina Kesika, Muruganantham Bharathi, Wipada Kunaviktikul, Areewan Klunklin, Chatnithit Chanthapoon, and Chaiyavat Chaiyasut. 2022. Essential Oils, Phytoncides, Aromachology and Aromatherapy—A Review. *Applied Sciences* 12, no. 9: 4495. https://doi.org/10.3390/app12094495

Aćimović, M., 2021. Essential oils: Inhalation Aromatherapy— A Comprehensive Review. *J. Agron. Technol.* Eng. Manag, 4, pp.547-557. https://www.researchgate.net/profile/Milica-Acimovic/publication/349485550_Essential_Oils_Inhalation_Aromatherapy_-A_Comprehensive_Review/links/6032d264a6fdcc37a84249c8/Essential-Oils-Inhalation-Aromatherapy-A-Comprehensive-Review.pdf

Passos, N.N, Campanelli, S. E; Silva C.R da; França R.C, da S; Nelson I.C. A. de S. R. Psychological and Neurophysiological Effects of Inhaled Aromatherapy. *Research, Society and*

Development, [S. l.], v. 11, n. 14, p. e442111436361, 2022. https://doi.org/10.33448/rsd-v11i14.36361.

Maddocks W. Aromatherapy in Nursing and Midwifery Practice: A Scoping Review of Published Studies Since 2005. *Journal of Holistic Nursing*. 2023;41(1):62-89. https://doi.org/10.1177/08980101221078736

Reflexology

Cai, Deng-Chuan, Ching-Yun Chen, and Ting-Yun Lo. 2023. Foot Reflexology: Recent Research Trends and Prospects. *Healthcare* 11, no. 1: 9. https://doi.org/10.3390/healthcare11010009

Huang H-C, Chen K-H, Kuo S-F, Chen I-H. Can foot reflexology be a complementary therapy for sleep disturbances? Evidence appraisal through a meta-analysis of randomized controlled trials. *J Adv Nurs*. 2021; 77: 1683–1697. https://doi.org/10.1111/jan.14699

Bach Flower Remedies

Porcar-Castell C, Esmel-Esmel N. The effect of Bach flower remedies on quality of life and sleep in hospital professionals during the Covid-19 pandemic. *TMR Integr Nurs*. 2021;5(6):195–202. https://doi.org/10.53388/TMRIN2021195202

Araújo Rocha M, Galvão Queiroz C, Gurgel Dos Santos KV, Dos Santos Dantas JK, Matias de Araujo SC, Ozorio Dutra SV, Vieira Dantas D, Neves Dantas RA. Bach Flower Remedies as Complementary Therapies in Health Care: A Scope Review. *Holist Nurs Pract.* 2022 Nov-Dec 01;36(6):E64-

E71. https://doi.org/10.1097/HNP.0000000000000552 PMID: 36255345.

Counselling

Sam J. Cooley, Ceri R. Jones, Arabella Kurtz, Noelle Robertson; 'Into the Wild': A meta-synthesis of talking therapy in natural outdoor spaces. *Clinical Psychology Review*,Volume 77, 2020, 101841, ISSN 0272-7358, https://doi.org/10.1016/j.cpr.2020.101841. https://www.sciencedirect.com/science/article/pii/S0272735820300295

Alison Brettle, Brettle Innovations Psychological therapies for depression A summary of the evidence. *Prepared for BACP November* 2012 Psychological therapies for depression: A summary of the evidence 2012 (pdf 0.3MB)

Reiki

McManus DE. Reiki Is Better Than Placebo and Has Broad Potential as a Complementary Health Therapy. *Journal of Evidence - Based Complementary & Alternative Medicine.* 2017;22(4):1051-1057. https://doi.org/10.1177/2156587217728644

Vanchenko, A. (2020). Positive impact of recreational techniques for the self-healing of the body. *Estudos de Psicologia* (Campinas), 37, e190082. http://dx.doi.org/10.1590/1982-0275202037e190082

COCOON

Ditch the News

Szabo, A., Hopkinson, K.L. Negative psychological effects of watching the news in the television: Relaxation or another intervention may be needed to buffer them. *Int. J. Behav.* Med.14, 57–62 (2007). https://doi.org/10.1007/BF03004169

Peace and Quiet

Melona C Deguma, Charisma G Lumayag, Mary Anne C Villaganas, Niña Rozanne T Delos Reyes, Jabin J Deguma, From anxious loneliness to meditation: a mental health self-care strategy to cope with the COVID-19 pandemic. *Journal of Public Health*, Volume 44, Issue 3, September 2022, Pages e402 e403 https://doi.org/10.1093/pubmed/fdab257

Bedtime Ritual

Lynch AM, Jarvis CI, DeBellis RJ, Morin AK. State of the Art Reviews: Nonpharmacologic Approaches for the Treatment of Insomnia. American *Journal of Lifestyle Medicine*. 2007;1(4):274-282 https://doi.org/10.1177/1559827607301397

Electronics/ Electro Magnetic Frequency EMF

Lear, R & Rees, C. (2025). *Safety of Wireless Technologies: The Scientific View.* 10.13140/RG.2.2.18625.06242

Levitt BB, Lai HC, Manville AM. Effects of non-ionizing electromagnetic fields on flora and fauna, Part 2 impacts: how species interact with natural and man-made EMF. *Rev Environ Health.* (2021) https://doi.org/10.1515/reveh-2021-0050

Yakymenko, I., Tsybulin, O., Sidorik, E., Henshel, D., Kyrylenko, O., & Kyrylenko, S. (2016). Oxidative mechanisms of biological activity of low-intensity radiofrequency radiation. *Electromagnetic Biology and Medicine*, 35(2), 186–202. https://doi.org/10.3109/15368378.2015.1043557

Carpenter David O, Bandara Priyanka Planetary electromagnetic pollution: it is time to assess its impact. *The Lancet Planetary Health:* Volume 2, Issue E512-E514, December 2018 https://doi.org/10.1016/S2542-5196(18)30221-3

An array of scientific articles and referenced research can be found on https://www.GBloc.co.uk https://www.gbloc.co.uk/post/recent-science-on-wireless-radiation.

CREATE

Shift the Focus

Kim, S. (2010). A Story of a Healing Relationship: The Person-Centered Approach in Expressive Arts Therapy. *Journal of Creativity in Mental Health*, 5(1), 93–98. https://doi.org/10.1080/15401381003627350

Vision On

Connellan, K. (2019). Dreaming, Healing and Imaginative Arts. Practice (1st ed.). Routledge. https://doi.org/10.4324/9781315199344

Darewych, O. H., & Riedel Bowers, N. (2018). Positive arts interventions: creative clinical tools promoting psychological well-being. *International Journal of Art Therapy*, 23(2), 62–69. https://doi.org/10.1080/17454832.2017.1378241

Colour Spectrum

Mantzio Michail, Giannou Kyriaki, (2018) When Did Coloring Books Become Mindful? Exploring the Effectiveness of a Novel Method of Mindfulness-Guided Instructions for Coloring Books to Increase Mindfulness and Decrease Anxiety Front. *Psychol.*, 30 January 2018 Sec. Cognition Volume 9 – 2018 https://doi.org/10.3389/fpsyg.2018.00056

Ashlock, L. E., Miller-Perrin, C., & Krumrei-Mancuso, E. (2018). The Effectiveness of Structured Coloring Activities for Anxiety Reduction. *Art Therapy,* 35(4), 195–201 https://doi.org/10.1080/07421656.2018.1540823

Elevate your Vibe

Jensen A, Bonde L. The Use of Arts Interventions for Mental Health and Wellbeing in Health Settings. *Perspectives in Public Health.* 2018;138(4):209-214. https://doi.org/10.1177/1757913918772602

MOVE
Affirm Up

Stephan, E., & Sedikides, C. (2024). Mental Time Travel as Self-Affirmation. *Personality and Social Psychology Review*, 28(2), 181-208. https://doi.org/10.1177/10888683231203143

Calm your Nerves

Bentley, Tanya G. K., Gina D'Andrea-Penna, Marina Rakic, Nick Arce, Michelle LaFaille, Rachel Berman, Katie Cooley, and Preston Sprimont. 2023. Breathing Practices for Stress and Anxiety Reduction: Conceptual Framework of Implementation Guidelines Based on a Systematic Review of the Published Literature. *Brain Sciences*13, no. 12: 1612. https://doi.org/10.3390/brainsci13121612

Feel the Sphere

Easwaran, K., Gopalasingam, Y., Green, D. D., Lach, V., Melnyk, J. A., Wan, C., & Bartlett, D. J. (2021). Effectiveness of Tai Chi for health promotion for adults with health conditions: a scoping review of Meta-analyses. *Disability and Rehabilitation,* 43(21), 2978–2989. https://doi.org/10.1080/09638288.2020.1725916

Ching Lan, Ssu-Yuan Chen, Jin-Shin Lai, Alice May-Kuen Wong, Tai Chi Chuan in Medicine and Health Promotion. *Evidence-Based Complementary and Alternative Medicine*, vol. 2013, Article ID 502131, 17 pages, 2013. https://doi.org/10.1155/2013/502131

Shake it Out

Klein, Penelope, George Picard, Joseph Baumgarden, and Roger Schneider. 2017. Meditative Movement, Energetic, and Physical Analyses of Three Qigong Exercises: Unification of Eastern and Western Mechanistic Exercise Theory. *Medicines* 4, no. 4: 69. https://doi.org/10.3390/medicines4040069

Letter It Go

Francis ME, Pennebaker JW. Putting Stress into Words: The Impact of Writing on Physiological, Absentee, and Self-Reported Emotional Well-Being Measures. *American Journal of Health Promotion.* 1992;6(4):280-287. doi:10.4278/0890-1171-6.4.280 https://doi.org/10.4278/0890-1171-6.4.280

Reading & Links

I have compiled a list of books that have helped me over the decades. At the time, some of these early books from the late 1980s and 1990s were crucial - this was before searching on the internet; I'm placing them here as I feel these are still relevant to this day. Research has moved on but the messages they share are core. In addition, I am including books that I have collected within my library over the last three decades that have been instrumental in my health restoration and maintenance along with others that you may find helpful to assist The Six Ways, you can find these in libraries, second hand/used bookstores online and offline along with possibilities of e-reader publications. The website links have been grouped in Ways for ease so you can begin to research and investigate. You will of course, discover your own and add to those you know and love.

Bach Edward Dr (2005) *The Essential Writings of Dr Edward Bach: The Twelve Healers and Heal Thyself.* Vermillion.
De Vries Jan (2003) *Treating Body, Mind and Soul: Alternative Solutions for Modern Living* Mainstream. Publishing
Dispenza Joe Dr (2019) *Becoming Supernatural: How Common People Are Doing the Uncommon*. Hay House.
Downing Dr Damien (1988) *Daylight Robbery: The Importance of Sunlight to Health.* Arrow Books
Downing Dr Damien, Dawes Dr Belinda (1989) *Why ME: a guide to combatting post viral illness.* Grafton
Dreamer Mountain Oriah (2000) *The Invitation. Element*
Emoto Masaru Dr (2007) *The Healing Power of Water. Hay* House UK
Farley Benjamin (2019) *The Unchained Life Manual: 16 Biohacks to Upgrade Body, Mind, and Spirit.* Independently Published.
Firstenberg Arthur, Souer Bob, (2020) *The Invisible Rainbow: The History of Electricity and Life.* Chelsea Green Publishing
Gibran Kahlil (1973) *The Prophet.* Knopf Publishing Group
Goddard Neville Hijazi Yann Editor (2003) *Neville Goddard - The Complete Collection - 12 books in 1*. Independently published
Hawkins David Dr (2020) *The Map of Consciousness Explained: A Proven Energy Scale to Actualize Your Ultimate Potential.* Hay House
Hay Louise (1985 2008) *You can Heal Your Life.* Hay House
Hay Louise (1991) *The Power is Within You.* Hay House
Jacobs Gill (1992) *Candida Albicans: Yeast and Your Health.* Optima
Lipton Bruce H (2015) *The Biology of Belief: Unleashing the Power of Consciousness, Matter & Miracles.* Hay House

Liberman Jacob (1990) *Light: Medicine of the Future: How We Can Use It to Heal Ourselves.* Bear and Co
Nestor James (2021) *Breath: The New Science of a Lost Art*. Penguin Life
McKusick Eileen Day (2021) *Electric Body, Electric Health: Using the Electromagnetism Within (and Around) You to Rewire, Recharge, and Raise Your Voltage.* Essentials
Murphy Joseph (2011) *The Power of Your Subconscious Mind.* Penguin
Myhill Sarah Dr and Robinson Craig (2024) *Diagnosis and Treatment of CFS ME and Long Covid, Third Edition; it's mitochondria not hypochondria.* Hammersmith Health Books
Norton Sally K Toxic (2023) *Superfoods: How Oxalate Overload Is Making You Sick—and How to Get Better.* Harmony/Rodale
O Becker Robert and Selden Gary (1998) *The Body Electric: Electromagnetism and the Foundation of Life*. William Morrow
Ober C, Sinatra S T, Zucker, M, (2014) *Earthing The Most Important Health Discovery Ever!* Basic Health Publications, Inc.
Penelope Ody (1993) *The Complete Home Herbal.* DK
Price Shirley (2000) *Practical Aromatherapy: How to use essential oils to restore health and vitality.* Thorsons
Roberts Kelly Rae (2008) *Taking Flight: Inspiration and Techniques to Give Your Creative Spirit Wings.* North Light Books
Robertson Robin (1992) *Beginner's Guide to Jungian Psychology.* Nicolas-Hays
Roytas Daniel (2024) *Can You Catch a Cold? Untold History & Human Experiments.* Humanely
Ruiz Miguel Don (2022) *Beyond Fear: A Toltec Guide to Freedom and Joy.* Chicago Review Press

Russell Stephen/Barefoot Doctor (1998) *Barefoot Doctor's Handbook for the Urban Warrior: Spiritual Survival Guide.* Piatkus

Russell Stephen /Barefoot Doctor (2004) *Barefoot Doctor Manifesto: The Internal Revolution.* Element

Russell Stephen/Barefoot Doctor (1999) *Barefoot Doctor's Handbook for Heroes: Spiritual Guide to Fame and Fortune.* Piatkus Books

Russell Stephen/ Barefoot Doctor (2002) *Liberation: The Perfect Holistic Antidote to Stress, Depression and Other Unhealthy States of Mind.* Element

Schauberger Viktor, Callum Coats (2000) *The Energy Evolution: Harnessing Free Energy from Nature (Schauberger's Ecotechnology).* Gill & Macmillan

Schwarz Joyce (2010) *The Vision Board.* Harper Paperbacks

Nenah Sylver, PhD (2021) T*he Rife Handbook of Frequency Therapy and Holistic Health: an integrated approach for cancer and other diseases.* 5th Edition, Second Printing

Singer Michael A (2007) *The Untethered Soul: The Journey Beyond Yourself.* New Harbinger

Steiner Rudolf (2008) *Spiritual Hierarchies and the Physical World: Zodiac, Planets and Cosmos: 110 Collected Works of Rudolf Steiner.* Steiner Books

Tisserand Maggie (1999) *Aromatherapy for Women: A Practical Guide to Essential Oils for Health and Beauty.* Healing Arts Press

Tolle Eckhart (2001) *The Power of Now.* Yellow Kite

Wilkinson Steve (1988) *ME and You: a Survivor's Guide to Post-Viral Fatigue Syndrome.* Thorsons

Zukav Gary (2022) *The Seat of the Soul: An Inspiring Vision of Humanity's Spiritual Destiny.* Ride

BOOST

www.allergyresearchgroup.com
www.ancientpurity.com
www.avogel.co.uk
www.fushiwellbeing.com
www.mercola.com
www.naturesplus.co.uk
www.riverford.co.uk
www.soilassociation.org

NOURISH

www.astonish.co.uk
www.earthing.com
www.faithinnature.co.uk
www.goodfoodproject.co.uk
www.groundology.co.uk
www.pan-uk.org/dirty-dozen
www.purdyandfigg.com/pages/about-us
www.waterdropfilter.co.uk

SUPPORT

www.absolute-aromas.com
www.aor.org.uk
www.bachcentre.com/en
www.bacp.co.uk
www.betterhelp.com
www.counselling-directory.org.uk
www.doterra.com/ME/en_ME
www.reikiassociation.net
www.therapy-directory.org.uk

COCOON

www.emf-protection.co.uk
www.gbloc.co.uk
www.headspace.com
www.insighttimer.com
www.nenahsylver.com/how-to-meditate
www.youtube.com/@MindAmend
www.youtube.com/@Delilahhelton

CREATE

www.augustwren.com
www.bethkempton.com
www.creativebug.com
www.creativelive.com
www.domestika.org
www.juliacameronlive.com
www.skillshare.com

MOVE

www.ddpyoga.com
www.headspace.com
www.pilateswithursula.com
www.psychologytoday.com/us/basics/affirmations
www.ruyischool.com
www.springforestqigong.com
www.tapwithbrad.mykajabi.com
www.taichisystem.com

About the Author

Julia Harvey is a Holistic Health Minder, Practitioner and Registered Counsellor. She has an Honours degree in Health from Liverpool John Moores University and certifications in Further Education Teaching, Spiritual Life Coaching, Reiki, Bach Flower Remedies, Animal Communication and Chakra Balancing. Recently, she has completed a Diploma in Clinical Supervision.

Suffering from debilitating ME in her twenties, Julia researched and studied numerous forms of complementary and integrative approaches to healing. She became her own holistic health investigator and has spent the past thirty plus years in educational and therapeutic settings, exploring the interconnectivity of health in all its modalities. Julia blends researched and intuitive health approaches with spirituality, coaching, energy psychology, and art, creating a holistic framework that nurtures the mind, body, and spirit.

She has a wealth of experience based around a broad range of issues from emotional health to physical health as well as a strong interest and thirst for knowledge relating to energy, vibration, frequency, and sound. Julia has continued to investigate and experience new healing methods and techniques and continues to share her knowledge with others, encouraging them to develop their own ReBalancing Toolkit.

In publishing her fourth book, The Way of the Boomerang, Julia's mission is to empower others to become their own holistic health investigator and practitioner, guiding them to rebalance their own health and self, and subsequently those around them in their community.

Other books by Julia

- Julia Harvey (2018) Muse Mantra Colouring Meditations
- Julia Dolowicz (2012) Creating your First CV in Seven Easy Steps
- Julia Dolowicz (2011) Writing your UCAS Personal Statement in Seven Easy Steps

If you'd like to receive my newsletter and hear about future books, workshops, upcoming podcast, education and training, please visit juliaharvey.co.uk to subscribe.

facebook.com/juliaharveyholistic
instagram.com/juliaharveyholistic
youtube.com/juliaharveyholistic
linkedin.com/in/juliaharveyholistic

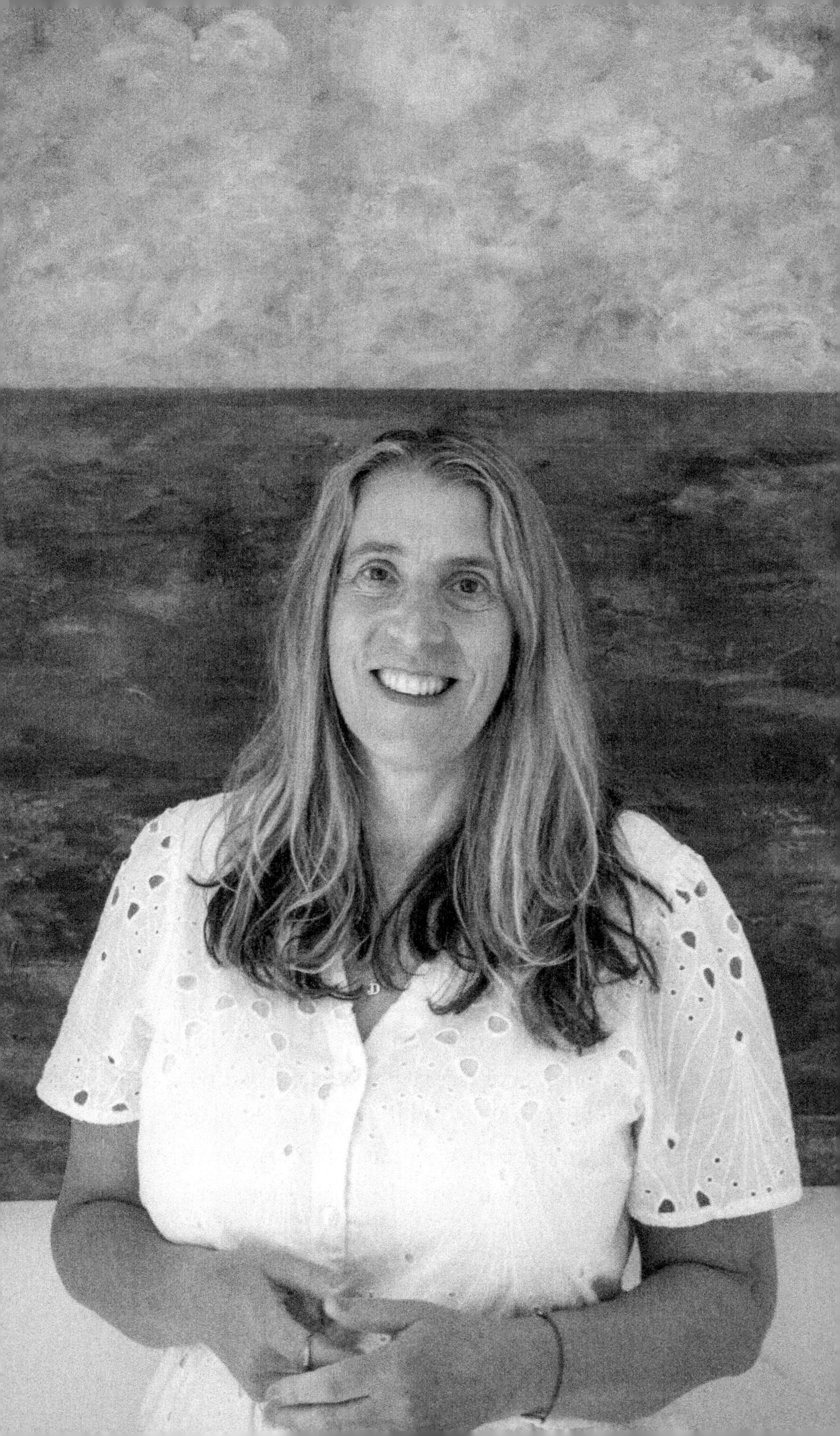

Myalgic Encephalomyelitis

Myalgic Encephalomyelitis (ME) is a long-term (chronic), fluctuating, neurological disease that causes symptoms affecting many body systems, more commonly the nervous and immune systems, affecting an estimated 250,000 people in the UK, and around 17 million people worldwide. People with ME experience debilitating pain, fatigue and a range of other symptoms associated with post-exertional malaise, the body and brain's inability to recover after expending even small amounts of energy.

According to Action for ME the causes of ME are still being investigated. Emerging evidence indicates that there are likely to be a number of factors involved and that there may be a number of different types or sub-groups of the illness.

There is evidence that certain infections can trigger the illness. Many are viruses but ME may be triggered in other ways.

Common viral triggers include glandular fever or Epstein-Barr virus (EBV). Other herpes viruses such as herpes simplex,

VZV (causes chickenpox/shingles), HHV-6 and CMV, may sometimes trigger ME, as can viral meningitis or labyrinthitis, commonly caused by enteroviruses, gastroenteritis, Hepatitis A, B and C infection, and in Australia, Ross River virus.

In a very small number of people, the trigger may have been an immunisation, given perhaps when they were already unwell, or a physical trauma, such as a road accident, operation, radiotherapy or chemotherapy, or whilst rare, it is suspected that a very few cases may be triggered by certain toxic substances.

One big outstanding question is whether emotional stressors can be a trigger. Studies are not clear, some suggesting a link and others not. It is very unlikely that stressful life events, such as bereavement, can trigger ME on their own.

Often it isn't possible to find out exactly what caused your illness – but you can still improve your symptoms, despite not knowing the exact trigger.

Not everyone will experience the same symptoms so it's important not to compare someone who has ME to another person who has the illness. People with ME can vary enormously in their experience of the illness, and also how long their symptoms last. Some make good progress and may recover, while others can remain ill for a number of years and may not get better. Some people find that they don't go back completely to the way they felt before they became ill, but they do recover sufficiently to lead happy and fulfilling lives. This is similar to many other chronic illnesses.

* Myalgic: meaning muscle

* Encephalo: meaning brain

* Pathy: meaning suffering or sickness

Symptoms may include persistent exhaustion (fatigue),

muscle and/or joint pain, sleep disturbance, flu-like symptoms such as headache, sore throat, painful lymph nodes, dizziness and/or nausea and problems with memory and concentration.

ME affects people in different ways and to varying degrees. It's a very fluctuating illness and symptoms can change over time. While it's important to find out more about the range of symptoms experienced by people with ME - it is also of value to know that people may only experience a few of them. Even in its so-called mildest form, ME can have a significant impact on an individual's life, and not just on their health. A lack of understanding and awareness about ME means patients can experience disbelief, and even discrimination, from friends, family, health and social care professionals and employers.

The National Institute for Health and Care Excellence (NICE) acknowledges that the physical symptoms of ME can be as disabling as multiple sclerosis, systemic lupus erythematous, rheumatoid arthritis, congestive heart failure and other chronic conditions. Other research shows that people with M.E. score lower overall on health-related quality of life tests than most other chronic conditions (Hvidberg et al, 2015)[2].

The October 2021 NICE guideline for M.E./CFS describes four levels of severity of ME/CFS, making it clear that "*individual symptoms vary widely in severity and people may have some symptoms more severely than others. The definitions below provide a guide to the level of impact of symptoms on everyday functioning.*"

These four levels of severity are :– mild, moderate, severe and very severe.

Mild: People with mild ME are mobile, can care for themselves and can do light domestic tasks with difficulty. Most are still working or in education, but to do this they have probably stopped all leisure and social pursuits. They often take days off, or use the weekend to cope with the rest of the week.

Moderate: People with moderate ME have reduced mobility and are restricted in all activities of daily living, although they may have peaks and troughs in their level of symptoms and ability to do activities. They have usually stopped work, school or college and need rest periods, often sleeping in the afternoon for 1 or 2 hours. Their sleep at night is generally poor quality and disturbed.

Severe: People with severe ME are unable to do any activity for themselves, or can carry out minimal daily tasks only (such as face washing, cleaning teeth). They have severe cognitive difficulties and depend on a wheelchair for mobility. They are often unable to leave the house, or have a severe and prolonged after effect if they do so. They may also spend most of their time in bed, and are often extreme.

Very severe: People with very severe ME are in bed all day and dependent on care. They need help with personal hygiene and eating, and are very sensitive to sensory stimuli. Some people may not be able to swallow and may need to be tube fed.

Source: www.actionforme.org.uk

Index

If not now, when?

Printed in Great Britain
by Amazon

60013758R00173